5-7 opt.

KID'S CHOICE
COOKBOOK

BY COLLEEN BARTLEY
& JOHN PATEMAN

<4 drink
juice or
milk
+ ½ ☐

>10 modify
next meal

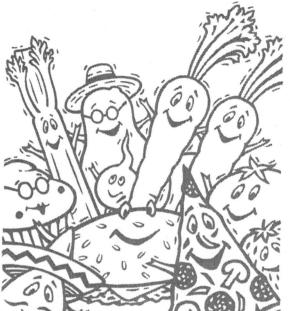

PICNICS Publishing
SECHELT, B.C., CANADA

KID'S CHOICE
COOKBOOK

BY COLLEEN BARTLEY
& JOHN PATEMAN

First Printing — October 1995
Second Printing — April 1997
Copyright © Colleen Bartley 1995

Canadian Cataloguing in Publication Data

Bartley, Colleen, date
      Kid's Choice Cookbook

Includes index.
ISBN 0-9680037-0-2

      1. Diabetes in children—Diet therapy—Recipes.
I. Pateman, John, date   II. Title.

RC662.B37 1995   641.5'6314   C95-900976-0

Published by PicNics Publishing
P.O. Box 2461, Sechelt
British Columbia, Canada
V0N 3A0
Fax: (604) 885-4375

Design:	Geoff Reed, Coast Creative Design & Advertising Ltd.
Illustration:	Tara Reed, Papyrus Design & Illustration
Typography:	Marianne Crocker

Printed and bound in Canada by Friesens Printers

TABLE OF CONTENTS

AUTHORS' ACKNOWLEDGEMENTS

We would like to thank all of the people whose support, confidence, and hard work enabled us to produce the "Kid's Choice Cookbook". A few 'behind-the-scenes' workers that we would especially like to thank are:

Doreen Yasui for her technical advice, her unflagging enthusiasm, and for her many hours spent reading the manuscript and checking our calculations.

Nancy Whitehead for her help in getting this project off the ground, and for always cheering us on.

Marianne Crocker for all of her hard work typing and editing.

Tara Reed for making our book come alive with her great illustrations.

Our children, Shannon, Heather, Megan, and Adam who helped test (and taste) the recipes and who are always an inspiration.

We would also like to thank our corporate sponsors, LifeScan Canada, Ltd.

DEDICATION

This book is dedicated to our mothers who taught us that "when life gives you lemons, make lemonade (sugar-free of course)!"

FOREWORD

At long last, a kid's "choice" cookbook! Parents will be happy to find it, kids will have fun with it. The recipes are just the kind of foods that kids love to eat.

Kids' Choice Cookbook recipes all include the Food Choice Values of the Canadian Diabetes Association so that they can easily be worked into a diabetic meal plan. The servings are generally smaller and fit with meal plans for young and school-age children. Many have been prepared and taste-tested by the author's daughter who has diabetes herself. All of the recipes will be enjoyed by each member of the family whether they have diabetes or not.

Colleen Bartley has combined her love of cooking with her years of experience planning and preparing meals (for her family and as a professional caterer with her partner John Pateman) to produce a creative and varied selection that will be helpful to many other families.

It is a pleasure for me to recommend this child-friendly "choice" cookbook to parents, caregivers, and most of all to kids with diabetes.

Have fun and enjoy the recipes everyday and for all those special occasions. I certainly will!

Doreen Yasui, RDN, CDE
Endocrine and Diabetes Service
British Columbia's Children's Hospital
Vancouver, B.C

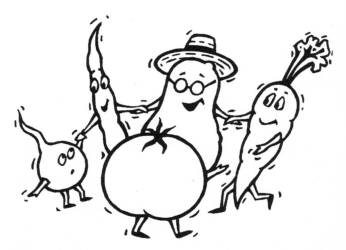

INTRODUCTION

Children with diabetes do not want to be set apart from other children by different eating habits. Parents want to provide nutritious food that kids will like. Parents also want to impress on their child at a young age the importance of following their meal plan. A regular balanced diet becomes essential when one has diabetes. With these challenges in mind it was our goal to develop a 'child-friendly' cookbook for children with diabetes.

It is also the Authors' belief that all children should be welcomed and encouraged in the kitchen. Establishing an early enjoyment of cooking can instill a lifelong confidence in an area that is so vital for good health. The recipes in this cookbook are written simply, with a minimum of fuss and ingredients. Some recipes are very simple which would appeal to young children as they can prepare the meal themselves. Other recipes are meant for cooks with more experience and sophisticated tastes.

In summary we hope that this book smooths the transition to a diabetic lifestyle by:
a) taking the emphasis off dietary restrictions by providing recipes that are familiar, tasty, and fun, and
b) encouraging a sense of freedom and control by letting kids prepare their own snacks and meals.

Before proceeding we would suggest that parents consider the following:

*Although each recipe has been analyzed for accuracy of food values, and is in keeping with the 1994 Good Health Eating Guide, meal planning should be done in conjunction with advice from your Dietitian. Nutritional analysis is based on the serving size stated on each recipe and symbolized with a happy face ☺.

* This cookbook is offered as a child-friendly collection of family favourites, adapted to a diabetic diet. However in keeping with our intent, the results can be enjoyed by everyone.

* The recipes in this book vary as to their degree of difficulty and thereby allow for increasing skill levels as the user gains experience. For first time cooks, have the child read through each recipe and gather all ingredients and materials before starting to cook. Keep the experience positive, encourage questions.

And please be aware that:

* Nutrient analysis was done using imperial measures, based on Bowe's and Church's 'Food Values of Portions Commonly Used' (16th. edition) and in the case of new products by using information from manufacturers and contained on manufacturers' labels.

* Unless otherwise stated, all recipes in this book were tested and analyzed using 2% milk, 0.1% yogurt, 1% cottage cheese, and partly skimmed (less than 20% M.F.) cheddar and mozzarella cheeses. 0.1% sour cream has recently been introduced into the marketplace in British Columbia and is used in this book as a suggested (optional) topping while 'light' (7%) sour cream was used in the actual development of the recipes.

* In some recipes, optional ingredients are suggested. These are NOT used in our calculations of Food Choice Values. If you are unsure as to how optional foods will affect Food Choice Values per serving, please ask your dietitian.

* The grams of carbohydrate in the Food Choice Values on some recipes may seem lower than the grams of carbohydrate stated in the recipe. This is because the grams of fibre have been subtracted from the total carbohydrates before Food Choice Values were calculated.

METRIC CONVERSION TABLES

CONVENTIONAL VOLUME MEASURE			CONVENTIONAL PANS		
1 ml	=	1/4 tsp	20 x20 cm	=	8 x 8 inch
2 ml	=	1/2 tsp	22 x22 cm	=	9 x 9 inch
5 ml	=	1 tsp	22 x 33 cm	=	9 x 13 inch
10 ml	=	2 tsp	25 x 38 cm	=	10 x 15 inch
15 ml	=	1 tbsp (3 tsp)	28 x 43 cm	=	11 x 17 inch
25 ml	=	2 tbsp			
45 ml	=	3 tbsp	20 x 5 cm	=	8 x 2 inch round
50 ml	=	1/4 cup	22 x 5 cm	=	9 x 2 inch round
75 ml	=	1/3 cup			
125 ml	=	1/2 cup	25 x 11 cm	=	10 x 4 1/2 tube
150 ml	=	2/3 cup			
175 ml	=	3/4 cup	20 x 10 x 7 cm	=	8 x 4 x 3 inch loaf
250 ml	=	1 cup	22 x 12 x 7 cm	=	9 x 5 3 inch loaf

COOKING TERMS AND TECHNIQUES

Beat: Make a smooth mixture by stirring vigorously with a fork, spoon, whisk or electric mixer.

Blend: Mix or stir two or more ingredients together to make a smooth mixture.

Boil: Cook a liquid over a high heat until bubbles rise to the surface.

Broil: Cook under "broiler" (top heating element) in the oven.

Chop: Cut into pieces with a sharp knife.

Coat: Cover or roll food in another ingredient.

Combine: Mix two or more ingredients together.

Dice: Cut into very small (5mm or 1/4 inch) squares.

Drain: Pour off or strain liquid from food.

Fold: Mix gently with a rubber scraper or spoon by lifting the bottom of the mixture outwards and over the top.

Fry: Cook in a open skillet.

Garnish: Decorate food with colourful additions such as parsley or fruit.

Grate: Rub food against a grater to make very small bits.

Grill: Broil under high heat or over hot coals.

Knead: Work dough by pressing and folding it with hands.

Marinate: Let food soak in a flavourful liquid.

Mince: Chop or cut into very tiny pieces.

Mix: Stir two or more ingredients together.

Pinch: A small amount of seasoning that you can hold between your thumb and forefinger.

Puree: Process or grind food into a smooth pulp in a food processor or blender.

Saute   (or Stir-fry): Cook in a skillet over medium to high heat while stirring constantly.

Season: Flavour food by sprinkling with herbs and spices.

Separate: Remove egg yolk from egg white before cooking.

Shred: Cut into very thin strips.

Simmer: Cook slowly at a low heat.

Stir: Mix with a spoon in a circular motion.

Toss: Mix food by lifting gently with salad tongs or two spoons.

Whisk: Beat or stir food with a wire "whisk".

Wok: A skillet especially designed for Chinese cooking.

BASIC RULES
FOR GOOD COOKS

MR. RADISH RULES

Before you start:

~ Wash your hands.
~ Read through your recipe carefully.
~ Make sure that you know how to use the stove and any other equipment you will need.
~ Be certain that you understand all of the instructions.
~ Place everything that you will need on the table or counter.

When you are cooking:

~ Measure everything carefully, choosing either the Metric or Imperial column for the entire recipe.
~ Always cut, peel, and chop downward and away from your body.
~ Have oven mitts handy when working with hot pans or dishes.
~ Always turn saucepan handles so that they don't stick out over the edge of the stove.

When you are done:

~ Make sure that the stove or oven is turned off.
~ Clean your work area.
~ Wash your dishes.

LET'S COMPARE

These are comparisons of food products (using the manufacturers' labels and the Bowes' and Church's 'Food Values of Portions Commonly Used - 16th. edition) that are available in the marketplace today. Keep comparing labels as new and healthier selections are developed.

	Carbohydrates	Proteins	Fats	Calories
Cheeses:				
30g or 1oz or 1/4 cup grated				
Cheddar	0.4	7.1	9.4	114
Low fat cheddar (40% less)	0.4	7.1	6.7	94
Part-skim mozzarella	0.8	6.9	4.5	72
Monterey Jack	0.2	6.9	8.6	106
Swiss	1.0	8.1	7.8	107
Cream cheese	0.8	2.1	9.9	99
'Light' cream cheese	1.8	2.9	4.7	62
1 cup cottage cheese (1%)	6.2	28	2.3	164
1 tablespoon parmesan cheese	0.2	2.1	1.5	23
Eggs:				
1 large egg	0.6	6.3	5.3	77
1 egg yolk	0.3	2.8	5.1	59
1 egg white	0.3	3.5	.2	18
Ice Cream:				
1/2 cup or 125 ml portion				
Regular ice cream	15.5	2.3	7.3	132
Regular Ice milk	15	2.5	2.8	92
1% ice milk	17	3.1	0.8	86
Frozen vanilla yogurt	15	2.3	2.9	104
Spreads: 1 tablespoon				
Butter	0	0.1	12.2	108
Margarine	0	0	11	100
Soft margarine	0.1	0	11.2	100
Soft diet margarine	0	0	5.6	49
Mayonnaise	0.1	0.2	11	100
'Light' mayonnaise	1.0	0.1	5.1	50
Miracle Whip 'light'	2.2	0.1	3.9	44
Mustard	0.3	0.2	0.2	4
Ground Meat:				
4oz raw / 3oz cooked				
Regular ground beef	0	21	18	248
Lean ground beef	0	21	15.9	233
Extra lean ground beef	0	22	14	219
Ground turkey	0	20.1	11.4	188

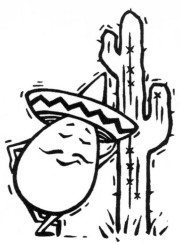

BREAKFASTS

Page		Carbohydrates	Proteins	Fats	Calories	Kilojoules
2	**Puffy Ham & Cheese Bake**	16	21	14	274	1151
3	**Mexican Scrambled Eggs**	15	13	8.5	192	806
4	**Eggs in Cereal Nests**	18	15	14	256	1075
5	**Crunchy French Toast**	51	14	8	328	1378
6	**Homemade Turkey Sausage**	3	13	5	111	466
7	**Breakfast Quesadillas**	16	16	9	207	869
8	**Pancake & Waffle Batter**	36	8	5	223	937
9	**Fun With Pancakes**	38	4	1	176	739
10	**Pancake Banana Split**	72	8	5	366	1537
11	**Apple Oat Pancakes**	43	5	1	201	844
11	**Apple Syrup (2tbsp)**	4	0	0	16	67
12	**Chocolate/Strawberry Waffles**	37	4	9	234	983
13	**Protein Plus Pancakes**	10	13	7	157	659
14	**Fruity Granola**	38	6	6	214	899

Nutritional Analysis (per Serving)

PUFFY HAM & CHEESE BAKE

4	Slices of whole wheat bread	4
15 ml	Soft 'diet' margarine	1 tbsp
250 ml	Grated cheese ('light' cheddar or Swiss)	1 cup
125 ml	Diced ham	1/2 cup
3	Large eggs	3
250 ml	2% milk	1 cup
2 ml	Salt	1/2 tsp
2 ml	Pepper	1/2 tsp
2 ml	Dijon mustard	1/2 tsp

☺ ☺ ☺ ☺ Makes 4 servings

1. Preheat the oven to 180° (350° F).
2. Cut the crusts off 3 slices of bread and spread both sides with margarine. Cut them into triangles and stand them up around the edges of a 20cm (8 inch) square baking dish.
3. Cut leftover crusts and remaining slice of bread into 1cm (1/2 inch) cubes and spread them on the bottom of the baking dish.
4. Mix the grated cheese and ham together and sprinkle over the bread cubes.
5. Beat the eggs, milk, mustard, salt, and pepper together; pour the mixture over the cheese and ham.
6. Bake at 180° (350° F) for 35 to 40 minutes, or until the eggs are set and the top is golden.

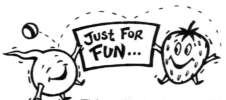

JUST FOR FUN...

This recipe is also good for brunch, lunch or supper. Try it with Hash Browns or Potato Pancakes.

Each serving: (1/4 recipe)

1	■	Starch choice
3	⊘	Protein choices
1	▲	Fats & Oils choice

MEXICAN SCRAMBLED EGGS

3	Large eggs	3
3	Egg whites	3
25 ml	2% milk	2 tbsp
2 ml	Salt	1/2 tsp
1 ml	Pepper	1/4 tsp
125 ml	Grated 'light' cheddar cheese	1/2 cup
50 ml	Chopped green onions	1/4 cup
50 ml	Chopped red or green peppers	1/4 cup
4 - 22 cm	Flour tortillas	4 - 8"

Optional Toppings: Salsa and 'no fat' sour cream

☺ ☺ ☺ ☺ Makes 4 servings

1. In a bowl, whisk the eggs and egg whites with the milk, salt and pepper.
2. Stir in the grated cheese, chopped green onions and peppers.
3. Wrap the tortillas in foil and warm in a 180° (350° F) oven for 5 minutes.
4. Spray a skillet lightly with vegetable oil spray and preheat to medium heat.
5. Pour in the egg mixture. Stir gently with a spatula and as the egg begins to set, lift the cooked portions and allow the uncooked portions to flow underneath until completely set.
6. Spoon the eggs into the centre of the warm tortillas. Fold over and serve with salsa and 'no fat' sour cream.

Did you know?

Light cheese is great melted!

Each serving: (1 tortilla)

1		Starch choice
1 1/2	⊘	Protein choices
1	▲	Fats & Oils choice

EGGS IN CEREAL NESTS

15 ml	Soft 'diet' margarine	1 tbsp
500 ml	Bran flakes	2 cups
175 ml	Grated 'light' cheddar cheese	3/4 cup
4	Eggs	4
	Salt and pepper (to taste)	

☺ ☺ ☺ ☺ Makes 4 servings

1. Using a microwave-safe bowl, melt the margarine in the microwave for about 30 seconds. Stir the bran flakes and grated cheese into the melted margarine.

2. Spoon the bran flake mixture into 4 small Pyrex baking dishes, making a 'well' in the centre of each one. Break an egg into the centre of each cereal 'nest'.

3. If microwaving: Poke each yolk with a tooth pick or a sharp knife point and microwave for 3 minutes on high (it takes less time if you are cooking only one dish at a time). OR

4. If oven baking: Don't poke the egg yolk. Simply cover the dishes with aluminum foil and bake in a 220° (425° F) oven for 10 to 12 minutes.

When poaching eggs in the microwave, always pierce the yolks first because, the pressure within the yolk as it cooks, could cause it to explode. Also, never microwave eggs in the shell.

Each serving: (1/4 recipe)

1	■	Starch choice
2	⊘	Protein choices
1	▲	Fats & Oils choice

CRUNCHY FRENCH TOAST

4	Eggs	4
125 ml	2% milk	1/2 cup
25 ml	Splenda®	2 tbsp
2 ml	Vanilla extract	1/2 tsp
1 ml	Salt	1/4 tsp
500 ml	Corn flake cereal	2 cups
8 slices	French bread, cut on the diagonal 1.5cm (1/2") thick	8
500 ml	Fresh strawberries	2 cups

Optional Toppings: Cool Whip® 'Light' and 'calorie reduced' strawberry syrup.

☺ ☺ ☺ ☺ Makes 4 servings

1. Spray a 25x38cm (10"x15") baking dish lightly with vegetable oil spray.
2. In a shallow bowl, such as a pie plate, combine the eggs, milk, Splenda®, vanilla and salt; mix well with a fork or a whisk.
3. Crush corn flakes by rolling between 2 sheets of wax paper with a rolling pin. Place the crushed cereal in another shallow bowl.
4. Dip the bread into the egg mixture, letting it absorb some of the liquid.
5. Dip the bread into the crumbs and place it in the prepared pan.
6. Freeze for 1 hour or overnight.
7. To serve: Preheat the oven to 220° (425°F). Bake the French toast for 10 minutes, flip and continue baking for 5 to 10 minutes. Serve with sliced strawberries, 'calorie reduced' strawberry syrup and a tablespoon of Cool Whip® 'Light', if desired.

This is a great choice for a special breakfast because it can be prepared the night before.

Each serving: (2 pieces)

2 1/2		Starch choices	1		Protein choice
1		Fruit & Vegetable choice	1		Fats & Oils choice

HOME MADE TURKEY SAUSAGE

25 ml	Minced onion	2 tbsp
45 ml	Quick rolled oats	3 tbsp
10 ml	Dried parsley	2 tsp
5 ml	Salt	1 tsp
2 ml	Ground sage	1/2 tsp
1 ml	Ground cloves	1/4 tsp
1 ml	Ground nutmeg	1/4 tsp
2 ml	Pepper	1/2 tsp
250 g	Ground turkey	1/2 lb
1	Egg white	1

☺ ☺ ☺ ☺ Makes 4 servings (8 patties)

1. In a small mixing bowl, combine the onion, oats, parsley, salt, sage, cloves, nutmeg and pepper.
2. In a medium mixing bowl beat the egg white with a fork and combine with the turkey. Add the onion and spice mixture and mix well.
3. Spray a large skillet with vegetable oil spray and preheat to medium heat.
4. Shape the turkey mixture into 8 patties and cook over medium heat for 12 to 15 minutes, turning once.

Each serving: (2 patties)

2	⊘	Protein choices
1	++	Extra choice

BREAKFAST QUESADILLAS

175 g	Turkey sausage (see page 6)	6 oz
4 - 22 cm	Flour tortillas	4 - 8"
50 ml	Salsa (recipe page 22)	1/4 cup
125 ml	Grated part skim mozzarella cheese	1/2 cup
50 ml	Chopped green onions	1/4 cup

☺ ☺ ☺ ☺ Makes 4 servings

1. Cook the turkey sausage, crumble. Set aside.
2. Preheat the oven to 200° (400°F). Spray a cookie sheet with vegetable oil spray.
3. Place 2 tortillas on the prepared cookie sheet, spread with the salsa, spoon on the cooked turkey sausage. Sprinkle with the cheese and the green onion. Top with the remaining tortillas.
4. Bake at 200° (400°F) for 6 to 8 minutes or until the cheese is melted and the edges begin to crisp. Cut each quesadilla in half and serve with extra salsa.

Each serving: (1 quesadilla)

1	■	Starch choice
2		Protein choices
1/2		Fats & Oils choice

PANCAKE AND WAFFLE BATTER

500 ml	All-purpose flour	2 cups
15 ml	Baking powder	1 tbsp
15 ml	Splenda®	1 tbsp
2 ml	Salt	1/2 tsp
125 ml	Plain 'no-fat' yogurt	1/2 cup
5 ml	Baking soda	1 tsp
375 ml	2% Milk	1 1/2 cups
2	Egg whites	2
5 ml	Vanilla extract	1 tsp
25 ml	Butter or margarine, melted	2 tbsp

☺ ☺ ☺ ☺ ☺ ☺ Makes 6 servings (12 pancakes)

1. In a large mixing bowl combine the flour, baking powder, Splenda® and salt.
2. In a measuring cup add the baking soda to the yogurt and let it foam.
3. In a small mixing bowl stir together the milk, egg whites, vanilla and melted butter (or margarine) until blended.
4. Add the yogurt mixture and the milk mixture to the flour mixture and stir until blended. Mixture should be thick and slightly lumpy; thin the batter with milk if it is too thick.
5. Lightly spray a large skillet or griddle with vegetable oil spray and preheat to medium.
6. Scoop 50ml (1/4 cup) pancake mix for each pancake onto the hot griddle. When bubbles on the surface of the pancakes start to pop and the edges are golden, turn the pancake and cook the other side.

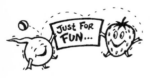 Add any of the following to the batter: 250 ml (1 cup) of blueberries, cranberries, fresh peach slices or sliced bananas and/or substitute 125 ml (1/2 cup) of the flour with oat bran, rolled oats, whole wheat flour or cornmeal.

Each serving: (2 Pancakes using the basic mix)

2	■	Starch choices
1	◆	2% Milk choice
1	▲	Fats & Oils choice

FUN WITH PANCAKES

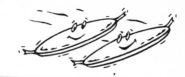

| 500 ml | Aunt Jemima® Complete Pancake Mix or, Complete Buttermilk Pancake Mix | 2 cups |
| 375 ml | Water | 1 1/2 cups |

☺ ☺ ☺ ☺ ☺ ☺ Makes 6 servings

For Teddy Bear Pancakes and Happy Face Pancakes use the above pancake mix.

TEDDY BEAR PANCAKES

1. Mix the batter following the directions on the package. Spray a griddle or a large skillet with a vegetable oil spray and preheat to medium-hot.
2   To form a teddy bear, pour 75 ml (1/3 cup) batter for the bear's body onto the hot griddle, then spoon on 25 ml (2 tbsp) for the head, and 5 ml (1 tsp) each for the ears, arms and legs; over-lapping the circles so it will stick together.
3. Cook until the edges begin to brown and bubbles appear on the surface, carefully flip and cook until golden. Decorate with raisins for eyes and nose. Serve with light syrup, if desired.

HAPPY FACE PANCAKES

1. Follow instructions in Step 1 above.
    Combine 75 ml (1/3 cup) of the batter with 2 ml (1/2 tsp) of cinnamon.
2   For each pancake, drizzle the cinnamon batter onto the hot griddle in the shape of eyes, nose, and mouth. Cook for 1 minute.
3. Pour 45 ml (3 tbsp) of the plain batter over each 'face'. Cook until the edges are done and the bubbles on the surface begin to break. Flip and continue cooking until golden. Serve with light syrup, if desired.

Each serving: (3 pancakes made with 45ml (3 tbsp) of prepared batter)

| 2 | | Starch choices |
| 1/2 | | Sugars choice |

PANCAKE BANANA SPLITS

500 ml	Aunt Jemima® Complete Pancake Mix or, Complete Buttermilk Pancake Mix	2 cups
375 ml	Water	1 1/2 cups
3	Bananas	3
500ml	Frozen strawberry yogurt	2 cups
375ml	Fruit (crushed pineapple, sliced strawberries, or blueberries)	1 1/2 cups

Optional:

75ml	'Calorie reduced' strawberry sundae topping	1/3 cup

☺ ☺ ☺ ☺ ☺ ☺ Makes 6 servings

1. Mix the batter following the directions on the package. Spray a griddle or a large skillet with a vegetable oil spray and preheat to medium-hot.
2. Scoop 45 ml (3 tbsp) of pancake mix for each pancake onto the hot griddle.
3. Cook until the edges begin to brown and bubbles appear on the surface, carefully flip and cook until golden.
4. To serve, place 3 pancakes on each plate. Top with 1/2 banana sliced lengthways and cut in half. Add 75 ml (1/3 cup) of frozen strawberry yogurt, and 50 ml (1/4 cup) of fruit such as crushed pineapple, sliced strawberries and/or blueberries and 15 ml (1 tbsp) of 'calorie reduced' strawberry sundae topping, if desired.

Pancakes become tough when flipped more than once.

Each serving: (1 pancake banana split made with 3 pancakes)

2 1/2	■	Starch choices	1	✳	Sugars choice
2	◢	Fruit & Vegetable choices	1	▲	Fats & Oils choice
1	◆	Skim milk choice			

APPLE OAT PANCAKES

75 ml	Quick rolled oats	1/3 cup
500 ml	Water	2 cups
500 ml	Aunt Jemima® Complete Buttermilk Pancake Mix	2 cups
125 ml	Grated apple (medium sized)	1/2 cup
25 ml	Splenda®	2 tbsp
2 ml	Cinnamon	1/2 tsp

☺ ☺ ☺ ☺ ☺ ☺ Makes 6 servings

1. Combine the rolled oats and the water in a medium-sized mixing bowl and let stand for 5 minutes.
2. Spray a large skillet or griddle with vegetable oil spray and preheat to medium-hot.
3. Add the pancake mix, grated apple, Splenda®, and cinnamon to the oats. Stir just until mixed (the batter will be thin).
4. For each pancake, pour 50 ml (1/4 cup) of batter onto the hot skillet. Cook until the edges look crisp and bubbles begin to break on the surface. Flip and continue to cook until golden.
5. Serve with light syrup or "apple syrup".

APPLE SYRUP:

Combine 175 ml (3/4 cup) unsweetened applesauce and 50 ml (1/4 cup) 'light' syrup in a small sauce pan. Heat over low heat and serve warm. (25ml [2 tbsp] = 1/2 sugars choice)

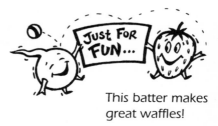

This batter makes great waffles!

Each serving: (2 pancakes)

2 1/2	■	Starch choices
1	**++**	Extra choice

CHOCOLATE & STRAWBERRY WAFFLES

500 ml	Aunt Jemima® Complete Waffle Mix	2 cups
50 ml	Unsweetened cocoa	1/4 cup
50 ml	Splenda®	1/4 cup
375 ml	Water	1 1/2 cups
750 ml	Sliced strawberries	3 cups
375 ml	Cool Whip 'Light'®	1 1/2 cups
6	Fresh strawberries for garnish	6

☺ ☺ ☺ ☺ ☺ ☺ Makes 6 servings

1. Preheat waffle iron.
2. In a medium-sized mixing bowl, combine the waffle mix, cocoa, and Splenda®; mix well.
3. Add the water and stir just until blended.
4. Bake in the hot waffle iron for 4 to 5 minutes or until steaming stops (or according to waffle iron instructions).
5. Serve topped with strawberries and Cool Whip® 'Light'. Makes 12 waffles.

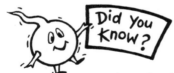

Aunt Jemima® Complete Pancake and Waffle mixes have very little fat. Hard to beat, even with home made mixes! Check out other labels.

Each serving: (2 waffles)

2		Starch choices
1/2	◆	Fruit & Vegetable choice
2	▲	Fat & Oils choices

PROTEIN PLUS PANCAKES

4	Eggs	4
250 ml	1% cottage cheese	1 cup
75 ml	All-purpose flour	1/3 cup
15 ml	Vegetable oil	3 tsp
2 ml	Salt	1/2 tsp

Optional Toppings: 'Light' pancake syrup or bananas and yogurt.

☺ ☺ ☺ ☺   Makes 4 servings

1. Beat the eggs in a medium-sized mixing bowl with a wooden spoon. Stir in the cottage cheese, the flour, 10 ml (2 tsp) oil and salt.
2. Heat the remaining 5 ml (1 tsp) oil in a large skillet, spoon in the batter (cook 4 at a time). Cook until both sides are golden brown.
3. Serve with 15 ml (1 tbsp) light pancake syrup or with 1/2 sliced banana and 1/4 cup yogurt. Makes 8 pancakes.

![Just for Fun...]

These pancakes can be frozen and reheated, making them a great breakfast choice for an active day (like a ski weekend)! To reheat, place the frozen pancakes in a single layer on a cookie sheet and bake at 180° (350°F) for 15 minutes.

Each serving: (2 pancakes)

1/2		Starch choice
2		Protein choices

FRUITY GRANOLA

575 ml	Quick rolled oats	2 1/3 cups
175 ml	Wheat germ (regular)	3/4 cup
75 ml	Flaked almonds	1/3 cup
75 ml	Honey	1/3 cup
50 ml	Splenda®	1/4 cup
15 ml	Vegetable oil	1 tbsp
15 ml	Water	1 tbsp
5 ml	Cinnamon	1 tsp
1 ml	Salt	1/4 tsp
75 ml	Pitted chopped dates	1/3 cup
125 ml	Raisins	1/2 cup
125 ml	Chopped dried apricots	1/2 cup
75 ml	Dried cherries or bananas	1/3 cup
50 ml	Hulled sunflower seeds	1/4 cup

☺ ☺ ☺ ☺ ☺ ☺
☺ ☺ ☺ ☺ ☺ ☺ Makes 12 servings

1. Preheat the oven to 180° (350°F).
2. In a large mixing bowl combine the oats, wheat germ, almonds, honey, Splenda®, oil, water, cinnamon, and salt.
3. Spread the oat mixture onto a baking sheet and bake for 15 minutes (until dark golden), stirring several times.
4. Immediately pack the hot mixture into a 2.5L (9" square) pan and let cool to room temperature.
5. When the oat mixture is cool, transfer it to a large mixing bowl and break it all into pea-sized pieces. Stir in the dates, raisins, apricots, cherries and the sunflower seeds.
6. Store in an air tight container.

Each serving: (125 ml (1/2 cup))

1	■ Starch choice	1/2		Protein choice
1 1/2	Fruit & Vegetable choices	1	▲	Fat & Oils choice
1/2	✳ Sugars choices			

BEVERAGES

Page		Carbohydrates	Proteins	Fats	Calories	Kilojoules
16	**Blender Breakfast Blast**	28	9	2	158	637
16	**Peach Nog**	18	11	3	141	592
17	**Peachy Banana Shake**	32	4	4	174	730
17	**Caribbean Shake**	29	1	0	118	496
18	**Frosty Strawberry Shake**	24	7	5	167	701
18	**Frosty Chocolate Shake**	27	7	6	181	760
19	**Old Fashioned Chocolate Soda**	24	5	5	156	655
20	**Iced Tea (Lemon)**	1	0	0	4	17
20	**Iced Tea (Spiced)**	5	0	0	20	84

Nutritional Analysis (per Serving)

POWER DRINKS FOR BREAKFAST

BLENDER BREAKFAST BLAST

1/2	Banana	1/2
125 ml	2% Milk	1/2 cup
125 ml	Plain 'no fat' yogurt	1/2 cup
50 ml	Wheat germ (regular)	1/4 cup
10 ml	Splenda®	2 tsp
250 ml	Frozen strawberries	1 cup

☺ ☺ Makes 2 servings

Combine the sliced banana, milk, yogurt and wheat germ in a blender or a food processor. Blend until smooth. Add the frozen strawberries and blend until frothy, about 1 minute. Sweeten with Splenda if desired. Serve immediately.

PEACH NOG

250 ml	Fresh or frozen peach slices	1 cup
125 ml	2% Milk	1/2 cup
125 ml	Plain 'no-fat' yogurt	1/2 cup
1	Egg	1
1	Egg white	1
10 ml	Splenda®	2 tsp
2 ml	Vanilla	1/2 tsp
1 ml	Nutmeg	1/4 tsp

☺ ☺ Makes 2 servings

Combine the peaches, milk, yogurt, eggs, Splenda®, and vanilla in a blender or a food processor. Process until smooth. Pour into glasses and sprinkle with nutmeg to serve.

BREAKFAST BLAST			**PEACH NOG**		
Each serving: (1/2 of recipe)			Each serving: (1/2 of recipe)		
2		Fruit & Vegetable	1		Fruit & Vegetable
1		2% Milk choice	1		2% Milk choice
1/2		Protein choice	1		Protein choice

FRUIT SHAKES

PEACHY BANANA SHAKE

1	Ripe peach, peeled and sliced	1
1/2	Banana, peeled and sliced	1/2
250 ml	Vanilla ice-milk (1%)	1 cup

☺ ☺ Makes 2 servings

Combine all of the ingredients in a blender or a food processor. Blend until smooth. Pour into 2 glasses and serve immediately.

CARIBBEAN SHAKE

1	Banana, peeled and sliced	1
125 ml	Pineapple juice	1/2 cup
125 ml	Orange juice	1/2 cup
250 ml	Ice cubes	1 cup

☺ ☺ Makes 2 servings

Combine banana slices and fruit juices in a blender or a food processor until smooth. Add ice cubes and blend for 1 minute. Pour into 2 glasses and serve immediately.

	PEACH BANANA			**CARIBBEAN**	
Each serving:	(1/2 of recipe)		Each serving:	(1/2 of recipe)	
1	◆ Fruit & Vegetable		3	◆ Fruit & Vegetable	
1/2	◆ 1% Milk choice				
1 1/2	✳ Sugars choices				
1/2	▲ Fats & Oils choice				

FROSTY MILK SHAKES

STRAWBERRY SHAKE

125 ml	Boiling water	1/2 cup
1	Package (10g) 'sugar-free' strawberry gelatin	1
500 ml	Vanilla ice milk (1%)	2 cups
250 ml	2% Milk	1 cup
125 ml	Ice cubes, crushed	1/2 cup

☺ ☺ ☺ ☺ Makes 4 servings

1. Pour the boiling water into a blender container or a food processor bowl.
2   Add the 'sugar free' strawberry gelatin. Blend at medium speed for 1 minute. Keep the blender running and add the ice milk by spoonfuls. Add the milk and ice.
3. Blend for 30 seconds. Pour into 4 glasses and serve immediately.

CHOCOLATE SHAKE

500 ml	Vanilla ice milk (1%)	2 cups
250 ml	2% Milk	1 cup
50 ml	Chocolate sauce (see recipe pg.107)	1/4 cup

☺ ☺ ☺ ☺ Makes 4 servings

1. In a blender, combine the ice milk, milk and chocolate syrup. Blend for 30 seconds. Pour into 4 glasses and serve immediately.

	STRAWBERRY			CHOCOLATE	
Each serving:	(1/4 of recipe)		Each serving:	(1/4 of recipe)	
1 1/2	◆	2% Milk choices	2	◆	2% Milk choices
1 1/2	✳	Sugars choices	1 1/2	✳	Sugars choices
1/2	▲	Fats & Oils choice	1/2	▲	Fats & Oils choice

OLD-FASHIONED CHOCOLATE SODA

10 ml	Unsweetened cocoa	2 tsp
15 ml	Splenda®	1 tbsp
25 ml	2% Milk	2 tbsp
125 ml	Vanilla ice milk (1%)	1/2 cup
	'Sugar free' Diet 7-Up®	

☺ Makes 1 serving

1. Mix the cocoa and Splenda® together in a tall glass. Add the milk and stir until completely blended. Spoon in the ice milk.
2. Slowly pour in the 'sugar free' Diet 7-Up®. Wait until some bubbles disappear and slowly keep adding the 'sugar free' Diet 7-Up®.
3. Serve immediately with a spoon and a straw.

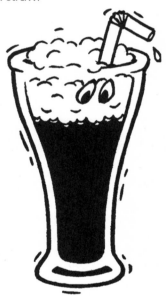

Each serving:

1		1% Milk choice
1 1/2		Sugars choices
1/2		Fats & Oils choice

ICED TEA

LEMON ICED TEA

1 1/2 L	Boiling water	6 cups
12	Tea bags	12
6	Lemon flavoured tea bags	6
125 ml	Splenda®	1/2 cup
2 1/4 L	Cold water	9 cups
1	Lemon, sliced	1

☺ ☺ ☺ ☺ ☺ ☺ ☺ ☺ ☺ ☺ ☺ ☺ ☺ ☺ ☺ Makes 15 servings

1.   Place tea bags in a large non-metal container. Pour the boiling water over the tea bags. Cover; and let steep for 6 or 7 minutes.
2.   Remove the tea bags and let cool.
3.   Stir in the Splenda® and the cold water. Serve over ice, garnish with lemon slices.

SPICED ICED TEA

5 ml	Whole cloves	1 tsp
8	Tea bags	8
1 L	Boiling water	4 cups
125 ml	Splenda®	1/2 cup
2 1/2 L	Cold water	10 cups
500 ml	Orange juice	2 cups
1	Lemon, sliced	1

☺ ☺ ☺ ☺ ☺ ☺ ☺ ☺ ☺ ☺ ☺ ☺ ☺ ☺ ☺ ☺ Makes 16 servings

1.   Place the cloves and tea bags in a large non-metal container. Pour the boiling water over the mixture. Cover; and let steep for 10 minutes.
2.   Remove the tea bags and cloves and let cool.
3.   Stir in the remaining ingredients. Serve over ice, garnish with lemon slices.

LEMON ICED TEA	SPICED ICED TEA
Each serving: (1 cup)	Each serving: (1 cup)
1 **++** Extra choice	1/2 ◆ Fruit & Vegetable

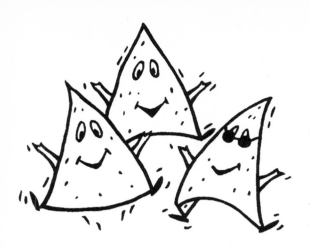

SNACKS

Page		Carbohydrates	Proteins	Fats	Calories	Kilojoules
22	**Salsa**	2	0	0	11	46
22	**Tortilla Chips**	17	2	3	105	441
23	**Guacamole Nachos**	21	7	14	235	987
24	**Potato Skins**	40	10	4	220	924
25	**Black Bean Dip**	8	3	2	60	252
26	**Hummus**	8	2	2	56	235
26	**Pita Chips**	17	3	2	96	403
27	**Mini Pizzas**	15	9	5	145	609
28	**Fast & Spicy Pizza Bagels**	27	10	8	222	932
29	**Quick Quesadillas**	15	9	5	139	584
30	**Tropical Peanut Butter Burritos**	32	6	11	236	991
31	**Buffalo Wings**	2	17	16	222	932
32	**Spicy Popcorn**	7	1	1	40	168

Nutritional Analysis (per Serving)

SALSA &
TORTILLA CHIPS

SALSA

175 ml	Diced tomato	3/4 cup
50 ml	Finely chopped onion	1/4 cup
15 ml	Chopped green pepper	1 tbsp
15 ml	Lime juice	1 tbsp
1	Clove garlic, minced	1
15 ml	Chopped parsley or cilantro	1 tbsp
5 ml	Minced jalapeno	1 tsp
	(or dash of hot sauce)	
2 ml	Chili powder	1/2 tsp
2 ml	Oregano	1/2 tsp
2 ml	Splenda®	1/2 tsp
2 ml	Salt & pepper	1/2 tsp

☺ ☺ ☺ ☺ ☺ ☺ ☺ ☺ Makes 8 servings

1. Stir all of the ingredients together in a small non-metal bowl.
2. Refrigerate to blend flavours for at least one hour. Salsa will keep in the refrigerator for up to 3 days.

TORTILLA CHIPS

8 - 22 cm	Flour tortillas	8 - 8"
	Vegetable oil or olive oil spray	
	Salt & Chili powder	

☺ ☺ ☺ ☺ ☺ ☺ ☺ ☺ Makes 8 servings

1. Preheat the oven to 200° (400°F). Lightly spray both sides of the tortillas with vegetable oil spray; sprinkle with salt and chili powder.
2. Cut each tortilla into 8 wedges. Place on a baking sheet; bake for 5 minutes. Serve with salsa and 'light' sour cream or guacamole if desired.

Each serving: **SALSA** (25 ml/2 tbsp)   Each serving: **CHIPS** (8 wedges)

1	**++**	Extra choice	1	■	Starch choice
			1/2	▲	Fats & Oils choice

GUACAMOLE NACHOS

140g	Unsalted nacho chips	5 oz.
250 ml	Grated part skim mozzarella cheese	1 cup
2	Green onions, minced	2
1	Large tomato, diced	1
1	Avocado, diced	1
1	Clove garlic, minced	1
15 ml	Chopped cilantro (optional)	1 tbsp
15 ml	Lemon juice	1 tbsp
1 ml	Hot sauce	1/4 tsp

☺ ☺ ☺ ☺ ☺ ☺ Makes 6 servings

1. Preheat oven to 180° (350°F).
2. For guacamole: In a small mixing bowl, combine the green onions, tomato, avocado, garlic, cilantro, lemon juice, and hot sauce.
3. Spread the chips in a single layer on a cookie sheet. Sprinkle half the cheese evenly over the chips. Bake at 180° (350°F) for 2-3 minutes.
4. Spoon 15ml (1 tbsp) of guacamole mixture onto each chip.
5. Sprinkle the remaining cheese evenly over the guacamole.
6. Return to the oven for 5 minutes, until the nachos are heated through.

Hard avocados can be ripened by burying them in flour for 1 or 2 days.

Each serving: (6 nachos)

| 1 | Starch choice | 1/2 | Protein choice |
| 1/2 | Fruit & Vegetable | 2 1/2 | Fats & Oils choices |

POTATO SKINS

6	Large russet potatoes	6
	Salt & Chili powder	
	Vegetable oil or olive oil spray	
250 ml	Salsa	1 cup
175 ml	Black beans (canned)	3/4 cup
125 ml	Frozen corn	1/2 cup
375 ml	Grated part skim mozzarella	1 1/2 cup
	(or 'light' cheddar)	

☺ ☺ ☺ ☺ ☺ ☺ ☺ ☺ Makes 8 servings

1. Preheat the oven to 200° (400°F).
2. Wash the potatoes thoroughly and pierce them with a sharp knife or a serving fork. Bake the potatoes on the oven rack until tender, about 45 minutes. Let them cool.
3. Cut the potatoes lengthways. Using a small spoon, scoop out all but 1cm (1/4 inch) of the potato. Be careful not to break the skin. Save the potato pulp for another use. Cut each shell into wedges.
4. Lightly spray the insides of the potato skins with vegetable oil spray; sprinkle with the salt and chili powder.
5. Move the oven rack 15-18cm (6-7") from the top element. Turn on the broiler.
6. Place the potato skins on a baking sheet, cut side up and broil for 5 minutes.
7. Combine the corn, black beans and salsa and spoon over the potato skins, dividing it evenly. Sprinkle with the grated cheese.
8. Return to the broiler and broil just until the cheese melts (3-4 minutes).

Each serving: (3 pieces)

2	■	Starch choices
1	◆	Fruit & Vegetable choice
1	●	Protein choice

BLACK BEAN DIP

1	Can (398 ml/14 oz) black beans	1
15 ml	Fresh lime juice	1 tbsp
50 ml	'Light' mayonnaise	1/4 cup
2 ml	Ground cumin	1/2 tsp
5 ml	Chili powder	1 tsp
50 ml	Diced red pepper	1/4 cup
15 ml	Diced jalapeno pepper	1 tbsp
15 ml	Chopped fresh cilantro (optional)	1 tbsp

☺ ☺ ☺ ☺ ☺
☺ ☺ ☺ ☺ ☺ Makes 10 servings

1. Combine the black beans, lime juice, mayonnaise, cumin and chili powder in a food processor and blend until chunky smooth.
2. Add the peppers and chopped cilantro, process until mixed but still a bit chunky.
3. Serve with tortilla chips or as a dip for fresh vegetables.

Each serving: (25 ml/2 tbsp)

Be careful when using jalapeno peppers. Some cooks use thin plastic gloves. Even the fumes can sting, don't rub your eyes!

1/2		Starch choice
1/2	⊘	Protein choice

HUMMUS
& PITA CHIPS

HUMMUS

1	Can (540 ml/19 oz) chick peas (garbanzo beans)	1
2	Cloves garlic, minced	2
25 ml	Lemon juice	2 tbsp
25 ml	Olive oil	2 tbsp
25 ml	'No-fat' yogurt	2 tbsp
2 ml	Salt	1/2 tsp
1 ml	Hot sauce	1/4 tsp
5 ml	Fresh dill	1 tsp
15 ml	Chopped fresh parsley	1 tbsp

☺ ☺ ☺ ☺ ☺ ☺ ☺ ☺
☺ ☺ ☺ ☺ ☺ ☺ ☺ ☺ Makes 16 servings

1. Drain and rinse the chick peas. Chop the dill and parsley and set aside.
2. Combine the chick peas, garlic, lemon juice, olive oil, yogurt, salt and hot sauce in a food processor and puree until smooth and fluffy.
3. Spoon in a shallow serving bowl. Smooth the top and sprinkle with the dill and parsley. Serve with pita chips and/or use as dip for raw vegetables. Makes about 500 ml (2 cups).

PITA CHIPS

1. Preheat oven to 180° (350°F). Cut 4-15cm (6") pitas in half to make 8 circles. Combine 15ml (1 tbsp) olive oil and 5ml (1 tsp) minced garlic in a small bowl and brush it on the outside surface of each pita round. Cut each round into four wedges. Arrange the wedges in a single layer on a baking sheet. Bake for 8-10 minutes, until golden. Makes 32 chips (8 servings).

Each serving: **HUMMUS** (25 ml/2 tbsp)   **PITA CHIPS** (4)

1/2		Starch choice		1		Starch choice
1/2		Fats & Oils choice		1/2		Fats & Oils choice

MINI PIZZAS

2	English muffins	2
25 ml	Pizza or spaghetti sauce	2 tbsp
125 ml	Grated part skim mozzarella cheese	1/2 cup
25 ml	Grated parmesan cheese	2 tbsp
2 ml	Italian seasoning	1/2 tsp
1 ml	Garlic powder	1/4 tsp
50 ml	Chopped ham OR 'light' cheddar	1/4 cup

☺ ☺ ☺ ☺ Makes 4 servings

1. Preheat the broiler with the oven rack 12-15cm (5-6") from the element (or use a toaster oven).
2. Mix the cheeses and Italian seasoning in a small bowl.
3. Cut the English muffins in half and toast under the broiler, cut side up, until golden.
4. Spread with pizza sauce. Sprinkle with garlic powder and top with cheese mixture.
5. Broil until the cheese melts.

JUST FOR FUN...

Experiment with your own favourite cheese and meat combinations...
Eg. shredded ham and Swiss with tomatoes, or wieners, cheddar and onions.

Each serving: (1 mini pizza)

1	■	Starch choice
1	⊘	Protein choice
1/2	▲	Fats & Oils choice

FAST & SPICY
PIZZA BAGELS

3	Bagels, split	3
50 ml	Pizza sauce	1/4 cup
6	Green pepper rings	6
6	Red pepper rings	6
6	Red onion slices (or to taste)	6
300 ml	Grated Monterey Jack cheese with jalapeno peppers	1 1/4 cups

☺ ☺ ☺ ☺ ☺ ☺ Makes 6 servings

1. Cut each bagel in half and spread each half lightly with pizza sauce.
2. Top with 1 slice of green pepper, 1 slice of red pepper and some red onion rings. Sprinkle each bagel with grated cheese.
3. Cook 3 bagels at a time on a microwave-safe dish covered with paper towels. Microwave on high for 1-2 minutes or until the cheese is melted and the bagel is hot.

Each serving: (1 pizza bagel)

1 1/2		Starch choices	1		Protein choice
1/2		Fruit & Vegetable choice	1		Fats & Oils choice

QUICK QUESADILLAS

2 - 22 cm	Flour tortillas	2 - 8"
15 ml	Salsa	1 tbsp
50 ml	Grated 'light' cheddar cheese or part skim mozzarella	1/4 cup
50 ml	Cottage cheese	1/4 cup
15 ml	Chopped green onion	1 tbsp

☺ ☺ Makes 2 servings

1. Place one tortilla on a microwave-safe plate.
2. Spread with salsa; sprinkle with the grated cheese and green onion. Spoon on cottage cheese. Top with second tortilla.
3. Microwave at medium-high for 1 minute or until the cheese is melted.
4. Cut into quarters and serve.

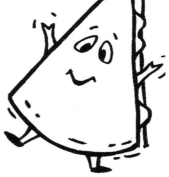

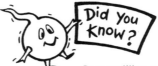

Quesadillas are good for breakfast or for an afternoon snack!

Each serving: (2 pieces)

1		Starch choice
1		Protein choice
1/2		Fats & Oils choice

TROPICAL
PEANUT BUTTER BURRITOS

4-22cm	Flour tortillas	4-8"
50 ml	Peanut butter	1/4 cup
50 ml	Crushed pineapple	1/4 cup
2	Bananas	2
50 ml	Coconut (unsweetened)	1/4 cup

☺ ☺ ☺ ☺ Makes 4 servings

1.   Spread 15ml (1 tbsp) of peanut butter along the middle of each tortilla.
2.   Drain the pineapple well and spoon 15 ml (1 tbsp) on top of the peanut butter.
3.   Slice the bananas thinly and divide evenly on the pineapple. Sprinkle the banana with coconut.
4.   Roll up each tortilla and serve immediately.

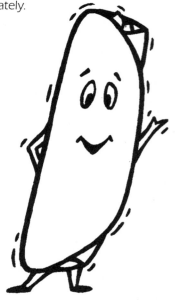

Each serving: (1 burrito)

| 1 | | Starch choices | 1/2 | ⊘ | Protein choice |
| 1 1/2 | ◣ | Fruit & Vegetable choice | 2 | ▲ | Fats & Oils choices |

BUFFALO WINGS

12	Chicken wings	12
25 ml	Soft 'diet' margarine	2 tbsp
25 ml	Hot pepper sauce	2 tbsp
5 ml	Paprika	1 tsp
2 ml	Salt	1/2 tsp
1 ml	Pepper	1/4 tsp

☺ ☺ ☺ ☺ ☺ ☺ Makes 6 servings

1. Rinse the chicken wings and pat dry with paper towels. Cut each wing into 3 pieces at the joints and discard the wing tips, leaving 24 pieces. Place in a shallow non-metal bowl.
2. Melt the margarine in the microwave for 60 seconds. Stir the hot pepper sauce and the paprika into the melted margarine.
3. Pour the margarine mixture over the wings. Stir to coat and refrigerate for 30 minutes or more.
4. Preheat the broiler with the broiler pan 18cm (7 1/2 - 8") from the element.
5. Arrange the chicken pieces on the rack of the broiler pan. Sprinkle with salt and pepper, brush with some of the sauce.
6. Broil for 20 minutes or until light brown.
7. Turn the pieces, baste with sauce and broil 10 minutes more or until tender and crisp.
8. Serve with 'fat-free' ranch or 'calorie-wise' blue cheese dressing as a dipping sauce.

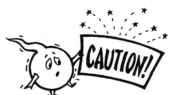

Each serving: (4 pieces)

Broiling fatty foods requires constant adult supervision!

2 1/2		Protein choices
2		Fats & Oils choices
1		Extra choice

SPICY POPCORN

125 ml	Popcorn kernels	1/2 cup
10 ml	Chili powder	2 tsp
5 ml	Vegetable oil	1 tsp
2 ml	Garlic powder	1/2 tsp
1 ml	Salt	1/4 tsp

☺ ☺ ☺ ☺ ☺ ☺ Makes 6 servings

1. Pop popcorn kernels in an air popper. Pour into a large serving bowl.
2. While the popcorn is popping, stir together the chili powder, vegetable oil, garlic and salt in a small bowl.
3. Gently stir the chili powder mixture into the hot popped corn. Stir until well coated.
4. Serve immediately.

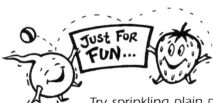

Just For FUN...

Try sprinkling plain popcorn with 25 ml (2 tbsp) parmesan cheese and 1/2 single serving size package of tomato soup mix.

Each serving:

1/2	■	Starch choice

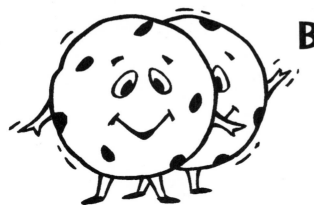

BAKING

Page		Carbohydrates	Proteins	Fats	Calories	Kilojoules
34	**Chocolate Chip Cookies (1)**	15	2	7	131	550
35	**Peanut Butter Cookies (2)**	15	3	7	133	559
36	**Oatmeal Shortbread (2)**	14	2	6	118	496
37	**Oatmeal Crunchies (2)**	16	2	5	119	500
38	**Peanut Butter Chip Cookies (2)**	16	4	7	145	609
39	**Applesauce Spice Cookies (2)**	17	2	6	125	525
40	**Rice Krispie Squares**	10	0	2	58	244
40	**Granola Krispie Squares**	13	1	3	81	340
41	**Chocolate Brownies**	8	2	5	80	336
42	**Peanut Butter Chip Muffins**	22	7	10	200	840
43	**Potato Cheese Muffins**	24	7	10	210	882
44	**Banana Bread**	33	6	12	257	1079

Nutritional Analysis (per Serving)

CHOCOLATE CHIP COOKIES

250 ml	Margarine	1 cup
125 ml	Brown sugar	1/2 cup
2	Eggs	2
25 ml	2% milk	2 tbsp
10 ml	Vanilla	2 tsp
500 ml	All-purpose flour	2 cups
250 ml	Splenda®	1 cup
5 ml	Baking soda	1 tsp
2 ml	Salt	1/2 tsp
575 ml	Rolled oats (Quick or old-fashioned)	2 1/3 cups
125 ml	Chocolate chips	1/2 cup

☺ ☺ ☺ ☺ ☺ ☺ ☺ ☺ ☺ ☺ ☺ ☺ ☺ ☺ ☺ ☺ ☺ ☺ Makes 36 servings
☺ ☺ ☺ ☺ ☺ ☺ ☺ ☺ ☺ ☺ ☺ ☺ ☺ ☺ ☺ ☺ ☺ ☺

1. Preheat the oven to 190° (375°F).
2. In a large mixing bowl, cream together the margarine and brown sugar (with an electric mixer or a wooden spoon), until light and fluffy.
3. Add the eggs, milk and vanilla, beat well.
4. In a separate bowl, stir together the flour, Splenda®, baking soda and salt. Add the flour mixture to the margarine mixture and mix well.
5. Stir in the oats and chocolate chips.
6. Drop by heaping teaspoonfuls onto an ungreased cookie sheet. Bake at 190° (375°F) for 10-12 minutes. Makes 36 cookies.

Splenda® does not have the preservative qualities of sugar so baking done with Splenda® should be refrigerated or frozen.

Each serving: (1 cookie)

1/2		Starch choice
1/2		Sugars choice
1 1/2		Fats & Oils choices

PEANUT BUTTER COOKIES

75 ml	Margarine	1/3 cup
125 ml	Brown sugar	1/2 cup
1	Egg	1
150 ml	'Light' peanut butter	2/3 cup
2 ml	Salt	1/2 tsp
2 ml	Baking soda	1/2 tsp
250 ml	All purpose flour	1 cup
125 ml	Splenda®	1/2 cup
2 ml	Vanilla	1/2 tsp

☺ ☺ ☺ ☺ ☺ ☺ ☺ ☺ ☺   Makes 18 servings
☺ ☺ ☺ ☺ ☺ ☺ ☺ ☺ ☺

1. Preheat the oven to 180° (350°F).
2. In a large mixing bowl, cream together the margarine and brown sugar (with an electric mixer or wooden spoon), until light and fluffy.
3. Mix in the egg, peanut butter, salt and baking soda.
4. Slowly blend in the flour and the Splenda®.
5. Add the vanilla and mix well.
6. Roll the dough into 36 small balls and place on a cookie sheet. Press flat with a floured fork.
7. Bake for 10-12 minutes.

Did you know?

When baking with Splenda®, stir it in with the flour instead of creaming it with the margarine as you would with regular sugar.

Each serving: (2 cookies)

| 1 | ■ | Starch choice |
| 1 | ▲ | Fats & Oils choices |

OATMEAL SHORTBREAD

175 ml	Butter, softened	3/4 cup
50 ml	Brown sugar	1/4 cup
50 ml	Granulated sugar	1/4 cup
5 ml	Vanilla	1 tsp
50 ml	Applesauce	1/4 cup
375 ml	All-purpose flour	1 1/2 cups
50 ml	Splenda®	1/4 cup
325 ml	Rolled oats	1 1/3 cups
	(Quick or old-fashioned)	
5 ml	Ground ginger	1 tsp
4 ml	Salt	3/4 tsp

☺ ☺ ☺ ☺ ☺ ☺ ☺ ☺ ☺ ☺
☺ ☺ ☺ ☺ ☺ ☺ ☺ ☺ ☺ ☺ ☺ ☺ ☺ ☺ ☺ Makes 25 servings

1. In a large mixing bowl, beat the butter with an electric mixer or wooden spoon until creamy.
2. Add the brown sugar and the granulated sugar, beat until light and fluffy. Stir in the vanilla and applesauce.
3. In a separate bowl, combine the flour, Splenda®, ginger, rolled oats and salt. Gradually blend the flour mixture into the butter mixture.
4. Press the dough into a ball and knead slightly until smooth.
5. Divide the dough in half; shape each half into a roll about 5cm (2") in diameter. Wrap the rolls in waxed paper and refrigerate until firm.
6. Preheat the oven to 150° (300°F).
7. Cut the chilled rolls of cookie dough into 50 6mm (1/4") slices and place on an ungreased cookie sheet. Bake at 150° (300°F) for 20 minutes.

Each serving: (2 cookies)

| 1 | ■ | Starch choice |
| 1 | ▲ | Fats & Oils choice |

OATMEAL CRUNCHIES

175 ml	Margarine	3/4 cup
250 ml	Brown sugar	1 cup
2	Eggs	2
5 ml	Vanilla	1 tsp
250 ml	All-purpose flour	1 cup
125 ml	Splenda®	1/2 cup
5 ml	Salt	1 tsp
2 ml	Baking Soda	1/2 tsp
650 ml	Quick rolled oats	2 2/3 cups

☺ ☺ ☺ ☺ ☺ ☺ ☺ ☺ ☺ ☺ ☺ ☺ ☺ ☺ ☺
☺ ☺ ☺ ☺ ☺ ☺ ☺ ☺ ☺ ☺ ☺ ☺ ☺ ☺ ☺ Makes 30 servings

1. Preheat the oven to 180° (350°F).
2. In a large mixing bowl, cream together the margarine and brown sugar (with an electric mixer or wooden spoon), until light and fluffy.
3. Add the eggs and vanilla, beat until smooth.
4. In a separate bowl, combine the flour, Splenda®, salt and baking soda.
5. Gradually blend the flour mixture into the margarine mixture. Mix well. Stir in the oatmeal (and raisins, if desired).
6. Drop by spoonfuls onto an ungreased cookie sheet. Bake at 180° (350°F) for 12-15 minutes. Makes 60

Optional: Add raisins, currants or dates.

Did you know?

When baking, always check the position of the oven rack before starting. You will have better results if you position the oven rack in the centre of the oven.

Each serving: (2 cookies)

1/2	■	Starch choice
1	✳	Sugars choice
1	▲	Fats & Oils choice

PEANUT BUTTER CHIP COOKIES

50 ml	Margarine	1/4 cup
50 ml	Brown sugar	1/4 cup
50 ml	Granulated sugar	1/4 cup
1	Egg	1
1	Egg white	1
125 ml	Peanut butter	1/2 cup
2 ml	Vanilla extract	1/2 tsp
375 ml	All-purpose flour	1 1/2 cup
50 ml	Splenda®	1/4 cup
2 ml	Salt	1/2 tsp
2 ml	Baking soda	1/2 tsp
125 ml	Quick or old fashioned rolled oats	1/2 cup
125 ml	Peanut butter chips	1/2 cup

☺ ☺ ☺ ☺ ☺ ☺ ☺ ☺ ☺ ☺ Makes 20 servings
☺ ☺ ☺ ☺ ☺ ☺ ☺ ☺ ☺ ☺

1. Preheat the oven to 180° (350°F).
2. In a large mixing bowl cream the margarine, brown sugar, and granulated sugar using an electric mixer or a wooden spoon, until light and fluffy.
3. Mix in the egg, egg white, peanut butter and vanilla.
4. In a separate mixing bowl, stir together the flour, Splenda®, salt, baking soda and rolled oats.
5. Add the flour mixture to the margarine mixture and mix well.
6. Stir in the peanut butter chips.
7. Roll into 40 small balls and place on an ungreased cookie sheet. Press the balls flat with a floured fork.
8. Bake at 180° (350°F) for 8-10 minutes.

Each serving: (2 cookies)

1	■	Starch choice
1 1/2	▲	Fats & Oils choices

APPLESAUCE SPICE COOKIES

125 ml	Margarine	3/4 cup
50 ml	Brown sugar	1/4 cup
1	Large egg	1
2 ml	Vanilla extract	1/2 tsp
300 ml	All-purpose flour	1 1/4 cup
125 ml	Splenda®	1/2 cup
5 ml	Baking powder	1 tsp
2 ml	Baking soda	1/2 tsp
5 ml	Pumpkin pie spice	1 tsp
1 ml	Salt	1/4 tsp
250 ml	Unsweetened applesauce	1 cup
325 ml	Quick or old fashioned rolled oats	1 1/3 cups
125 ml	Currants or raisins	1/2 cup

☺ ☺ ☺ ☺ ☺ ☺ ☺ ☺ ☺ ☺ Makes 20 servings
☺ ☺ ☺ ☺ ☺ ☺ ☺ ☺ ☺ ☺

1. Preheat the oven to 180° (350°F).
2. In a large mixing bowl, cream together the margarine and brown sugar, using an electric mixer or a wooden spoon, until light and fluffy.
3. Add the egg, and vanilla, mix well
4. In a separate bowl, stir together the flour, Splenda®, baking powder, baking soda, pumpkin pie spice and salt.
5. Add the flour mixture and the applesauce gradually to the margarine mixture and mix well.
6. Stir in the rolled oats and currants.
7. Drop by teaspoonfuls onto a cookie sheet, making 40 cookies. Bake at 180° (350°F) for 12-15 minutes.

Each serving: (2 cookies)

1	■	Starch choice
1	▲	Fats & Oils choice

RICE KRISPIE SQUARES

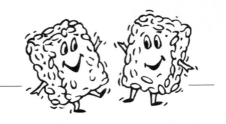

RICE KRISPIE SQUARES:

50 ml	Margarine	1/4 cup
750 ml	Mini marshmallows	3 cups
5 ml	Vanilla	1 tsp
1250 ml	Rice Krispies®	5 cups

☺ ☺ ☺ ☺ ☺ ☺ ☺ ☺ ☺ ☺ ☺ ☺ Makes 24 servings
☺ ☺ ☺ ☺ ☺ ☺ ☺ ☺ ☺ ☺ ☺ ☺

1. Melt the margarine in a large heavy saucepan.
2   Add the marshmallows and stir over low heat until the marshmallows are melted.
3. Remove from the heat and stir in the vanilla and Rice Krispies®. Mix until evenly coated.
4. Spoon into a 23cm (9") square pan. Moisten your hands with cold water and press the Rice Krispie® mixture firmly and evenly into the pan.
5. Refrigerate for 30 minutes or more. Cut into 24 squares.

Note: "Reprinted from Choice Cooking, copyright 1982, with permission from the Canadian Diabetes Association"

GRANOLA KRISPIE SQUARES:

| 75 ml each | Rolled oats and flaked unsweetened coconut | 1/3 cup each |
| 50 ml each | Cocoa, raisins and chocolate chips | 1/4 cup each |

1. Complete steps 1 through 3 above. Add the coconut, raisins, chocolate chips and rolled oats. Mix until evenly coated.
2   Press into a 3.5L (9"x13") pan.
3. Refrigerate for 30 minutes or more. Cut into 24 squares.

	RICE KRISPIE®			**GRANOLA KRISPIE**	
Each serving: (1 square)			Each serving: (1 square)		
1	✳	Sugars choice	1/2	◼	Starch choice
1/2	▲	Fats & Oils choice	1/2	✳	Sugars choice
			1/2	▲	Fats & Oils choice

CHOCOLATE BROWNIES

125 ml	Splenda®	1/2 cup
150 ml	All-purpose flour	2/3 cup
75 ml	Unsweetened cocoa powder	1/3 cup
5 ml	Baking powder	1 tsp
1 ml	Salt	1/4 tsp
75 ml	Soft 'diet' margarine	1/3 cup
2	Eggs	2
5 ml	Vanilla	1 tsp
125 ml	Unsweetened applesauce	1/2 cup
75 ml	Chopped walnuts 50g (2 oz.)	1/3 cup

☺ ☺ ☺ ☺ ☺ ☺ ☺ ☺ Makes 16 servings
☺ ☺ ☺ ☺ ☺ ☺ ☺ ☺

1. Preheat the oven to 180° (350°F). Spray a 2L (8" square) cake pan with vegetable oil spray and set aside.
2. In a medium-sized bowl, stir together the flour, Splenda®, cocoa, baking powder and salt with a wooden spoon. Stir in walnuts and set aside.
3. With an electric mixer, beat the margarine, eggs, and vanilla for 1 minute. Add the applesauce and beat just until blended.
4. Add the flour mixture to the egg mixture and stir on low speed just until moistened.
5. Spread batter evenly into the prepared cake pan. Bake at 180° (350°F) for 15 minutes. Remove from the oven and insert a toothpick into the centre of the brownies, if it comes out clean, they are done! Cut into 16 squares before serving.

Did You Know?

Unsweetened cocoa powder has only 115 calories and 4 grams of fat in 75ml (1/3 cup), whereas 25g (1 oz) of unsweetened baking chocolate has 139 calories and 14 grams of fat.

Each serving: (1 brownie)

| 1/2 | | Starch choice |
| 1 | | Fats & Oils choice |

PEANUT BUTTER CHIP MUFFINS

375 ml	Whole wheat flour	1 1/2 cups
300 ml	Quick rolled oats	1 1/4 cups
50 ml	Wheat germ (regular)	1/4 cup
125 ml	Splenda®	1/2 cup
20 ml	Baking powder	4 tsp
5 ml	Baking soda	1 tsp
5 ml	Salt and vanilla	1 tsp
75 ml	Chocolate chips	1/3 cup
250 ml	Plain 'no-fat' yogurt	1 cup
25 ml	Liquid honey	2 tbsp
125 ml	Peanut butter	1/2 cup
50 ml	Vegetable oil	1/4 cup
2	Eggs	2
1	Egg white	1
5 ml	Vanilla	1 tsp

☺ ☺ ☺ ☺ ☺ ☺ ☺ ☺ ☺ ☺ ☺ ☺ ☺ ☺ ☺ Makes 15 servings

1. Preheat the oven to 190° (375°F). Line muffin tins with paper cups (or spray with vegetable oil spray).
2. In a large mixing bowl, stir together the flour, oats, wheat germ, Splenda®, baking powder, baking soda, and salt. Stir in the chocolate chips and set aside.
3. In a separate bowl, beat together the yogurt, honey, peanut butter, oil, eggs, egg white and vanilla. Beat until smooth.
4. Add the flour mixture to the yogurt mixture and stir JUST until mixed.
5. Spoon the batter into the paper lined muffin tins and bake at 190° (375°F) for 25-30 minutes, or until firm.

Each serving: (1 muffin)

1	■	Starch choices	1/2		Protein choice
1/2	✳	Sugars choice	1 1/2	▲	Fats & Oils choice

Page 42

POTATO CHEESE MUFFINS

500 ml	All purpose flour	2 cups
75 ml	Splenda®	1/3 cup
20 ml	Baking powder	4 tsp
5 ml	Salt	1 tsp
2	Eggs	2
375 ml	2% Milk	1 1/2 cups
125 ml	Cooked mashed potatoes	1/2 cup
175 ml	Grated 'light' Cheddar cheese	3/4 cup
75 ml	Margarine, melted	1/3 cup

☺ ☺ ☺ ☺ ☺ ☺ ☺ ☺ ☺ ☺ Makes 10 servings

1. Preheat the oven to 200° (400°F). Line 10 muffin tins with paper cups (or spray with vegetable oil spray).
2. In a large mixing bowl, combine the flour, Splenda®, baking powder and salt.
3. In a medium-sized mixing bowl, beat the eggs well with an electric mixer or a wooden spoon.
4. Stir in the milk, mashed potatoes, grated cheese, and melted margarine. Mix well.
5. Add the egg mixture to the flour mixture and stir just until mixed.
6. Spoon the batter into the paper lined muffin tins and bake at 200° (400°F) for 25 minutes, or until firm and lightly browned.

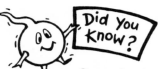

Over-mixed muffin batter will make the muffins tough, flat topped, and full of tunnels. The rule is to stir 20 times (with a wooden spoon) when you have added the flour mixture to the egg mixture.

Each serving: (1 muffin)

1 1/2		Starch choices
1/2		Protein choice
1 1/2		Fats & Oils choices

BANANA BREAD

2	Eggs	2
50 ml	Brown sugar	1/4 cup
50 ml	Vegetable oil	1/4 cup
250 ml	Mashed ripe bananas	1 cup
50 ml	Unsweetened applesauce	1/4 cup
500 ml	All purpose flour	2 cups
125 ml	Splenda®	1/2 cup
5 ml	Baking powder	1 tsp
5 ml	Baking soda	1 tsp
2 ml	Salt	1/2 tsp
125 ml	Chopped walnuts	1/2 cup

☺ ☺ ☺ ☺ ☺ ☺ ☺ ☺ ☺ ☺ Makes 10 servings

1. Preheat the oven to 180° (350°F). Spray a 1.5L loaf pan with vegetable oil spray and dust with flour.
2. Beat the eggs, brown sugar, oil, bananas and applesauce with an electric beater or wooden spoon, until well mixed.
3. In a separate bowl, mix together the flour, Splenda®, baking powder, baking soda, and salt.
4. Add the flour mixture to the egg mixture and stir, just until combined.
5. Pour the batter into the prepared loaf pan. Bake for 55-60 minutes or until a toothpick inserted in the centre comes out clean.
6. Let cool for 15 minutes, then turn out onto a wire rack to cool completely.

Each serving: (1/10 recipe)

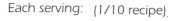

2		Starch choices
1/2		Fruit & Vegetable choice
2 1/2		Fats & Oils choices

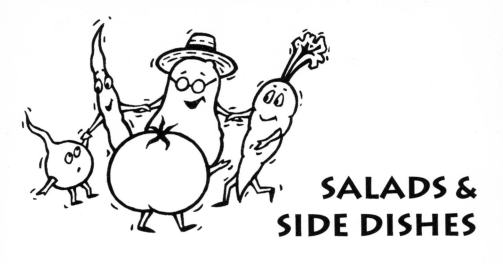

SALADS & SIDE DISHES

Nutritional Analysis (per Serving)

FRIED RICE

750 ml	Cooked rice (cooled)	3 cups
10 ml	Vegetable oil	2 tsp
3	Eggs	3
125 ml	Grated carrots	1/2 cup
50 ml	Chopped celery	1/4 cup
125 ml	Sliced mushrooms	1/2 cup
50 ml	Sliced green onions	1/4 cup
125 ml	Frozen peas	1/2 cup
125 ml	Cooked meat eg., shrimp, ham or chicken (chopped)	1/2 cup
45 ml	Soy sauce (low sodium)	3 tbsp

☺ ☺ ☺ ☺ ☺ ☺ Makes 6 servings

1. In a wok or a large non-stick skillet, heat 5 ml (1 tsp) of the oil over medium heat.
2. Beat the eggs with a fork. Cook and stir in the wok until scrambled. Remove from pan and cut into thin strips. Set aside.
3. In the same pan, heat the remaining 5 ml (1 tsp) of oil and saute the carrots, celery, and mushrooms for 5 minutes or until the mushrooms are soft.
4. Stir in the green onions and cook for 1 minute.
5. Add the peas, meat and rice. Sprinkle with soy sauce and toss gently. Stir in the scrambled eggs.
6. Cover and cook 3-4 minutes or until heated through.

Each serving: (1/6 recipe)

| 2 | Starch choices | 1 | Protein choice |
| 1/2 | Fruit & Vegetable choice | 1/2 | Fats & Oils choice |

OVEN FRENCH FRIES

1 kg	4 Large baking potatoes	2 lbs
20 ml	Vegetable oil	4 tsp
	Salt or seasoned salt	

☺ ☺ ☺ ☺ ☺ ☺ Makes 6 servings

1. Peel the potatoes and cut lengthways into 1cm (1/4 inch) strips. Soak in cold water for 15 minutes or longer. Drain and pat dry with paper towels.
2. Preheat the oven to 230° (450°F). Spray a baking pan thoroughly with vegetable oil spray.
3. Place the potato strips on the baking pan and toss with the vegetable oil to coat evenly. Spread the potatoes into a single layer.
4. Bake at 230° (450°F) for 20 minutes. Turn potatoes and continue baking for 15 minutes or until crisp and golden.
5. Sprinkle with salt and serve.

Variations:

Parmesan Potatoes: Cut the potatoes into 1cm (1/4 inch) thick strips. Proceed as above but after turning, sprinkle lightly with parmesan cheese.

Herb Potatoes: Bake 30 minutes, as above. Then sprinkle with 15 ml (1 tbsp) fresh chopped parsley, one clove minced garlic and salt, toss. Bake 5 minutes more.

Each serving: (1/6 recipe)

1 1/2		Starch choices
1/2		Fats & Oils choice

MASHED POTATO CASSEROLE

1 kg	6 medium potatoes	2 lbs
15 ml	Soft 'diet' margarine	1 tbsp
125 ml	1% cottage cheese	1/2 cup
2	Eggs	2
175 ml	Grated 'light' cheddar cheese	3/4 cup
50 ml	'Light' sour cream	1/4 cup
2 ml	Salt	1/2 tsp
1 ml	Pepper	1/4 tsp
Pinch	Nutmeg	Pinch

☺ ☺ ☺ ☺ ☺ ☺ Makes 6 servings

1. Peel the potatoes and cut into quarters. Put into a medium sized saucepan. Add just enough water to cover the potatoes and add 5 ml (1 tsp) of salt. Bring to a boil, lower heat to simmer, cover saucepan and let simmer until potatoes are tender (about 20 minutes). Drain well.
2   Mash potatoes with a potato masher and mix in the margarine.
3. Puree the cottage cheese and eggs in a food processor or blender. Stir into the potatoes. Add the cheddar cheese, sour cream and spices, mix well.
4. Spray a 1.5L (6 cup) casserole with vegetable oil spray and spoon in the potato mixture. Bake, uncovered at 200° (400°F) for 20-25 minutes.

Did You Know?

This recipe can be made early in the day and baked at supper time.

Each serving: (1/6 recipe)

2		Starch choices
1		Protein choice
1		Fats & Oils choice

STUFFED BAKED POTATOES

4 medium	Baking potatoes	4 medium
50 ml	1% cottage cheese	1/4 cup
25 ml	Minced chives or green onions	2 tbsp
25 ml	Plain 'no-fat' yogurt	2 tbsp
2 ml	Salt	1/2 tsp
1 ml	Pepper	1/4 tsp
50 ml	Grated part skim mozzarella or 'light' cheddar cheese	1/4 cup

☺ ☺ ☺ ☺ Makes 4 servings

1. Preheat the oven to 200° (400°F).
2. Wash and scrub the potatoes well. Dry with paper towels. Pierce each potato with a large fork and bake for 50 to 60 minutes, or until tender. Let cool.
3. Reduce oven temperature to 180° (350°F).
4. Split the potatoes in half lengthways and using a small spoon, scoop out the potato, leaving the skin intact.
5. Place the potato pulp in a medium-sized mixing bowl. Add the cottage cheese, minced green onions, yogurt, salt and pepper. Mash with a fork and spoon back into the potato skins.
6. Place the potatoes in a shallow baking dish and top each one with 15 ml (1 tbsp) of grated cheese.
7. Return the potatoes to the oven and bake for 15 minutes.

Each serving: (1 potato)

2		Starch choices
1/2		Protein choice

POTATO PANCAKES

4	Medium potatoes	4
125 ml	Grated carrots	1/2 cup
25 ml	Grated onion	2 tbsp
75 ml	Flour	1/3 cup
5 ml	Salt	1 tsp
2 ml	Baking powder	1/2 tsp
75 ml	2% milk	1/3 cup
2	Eggs	2
25 ml	Vegetable oil	2 tbsp
125 ml	Unsweetened applesauce	1/2 cup
125 ml	'Light' sour cream	1/2 cup

☺ ☺ ☺ ☺ Makes 4 servings

1. Peel the potatoes and cut them in half. Put them into a saucepan, add just enough water to cover, bring to a boil and then simmer until tender (about 20 minutes). Drain and let cool.
2. Grate the potatoes (you should have 500ml [2 cups]), carrots, and onions and combine in a medium-sized mixing bowl.
3. Stir together the flour, baking powder and salt. Pour over the potatoes and toss with a fork to mix.
4. Combine the eggs and milk and stir into the potato mixture.
5. Heat 15 ml (1 tbsp) of vegetable oil in a large skillet. Using 1/2 of the batter, scoop four mounds into the preheated pan. Flatten each mound to 1cm (1/2") with a metal spatula. Fry until deep brown on both sides, turning only once.
6. Remove pancakes and place on paper towels. Add the remaining 15ml (1 tbsp) of oil to skillet. Repeat with the remaining batter.
7. Best served hot from the skillet. Top with unsweetened apple sauce and 'light' sour cream.

Each serving: (2 pancakes)

2	■	Starch choices	1/2		Protein choice
1/2		Fruit & Vegetable choice	2		Fats & Oils choices

CORN ON THE COB

6	Cobs of corn	6
	Flavoured butters:	
45 ml	Soft 'diet' margarine	3 tbsp
2 ml	Salt	1/2 tsp
1 ml	Pepper	1/4 tsp
15 ml	Minced green onion or	1 tbsp
15 ml	Chopped parsley or	1 tbsp
2 ml	Chili powder	1/2 tsp

☺ ☺ ☺ ☺ ☺ ☺ Makes 6 servings

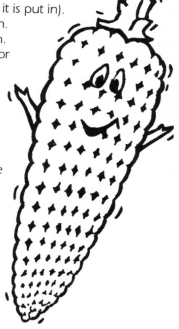

1. Bring to a boil, a large saucepan of salted water (enough water to cover the corn when it is put in).
2. Remove the husks and silk from the corn.
3. When the water is boiling, add the corn. Reduce the heat to medium and cook for 4-5 minutes.
4. Drain the corn and serve with your choice of flavoured butters.

FLAVOURED BUTTER

While corn is cooking, combine soft margarine with salt, pepper, and your choice of herb or spice. (Try it sprinkled with parmesan cheese, 5 ml [1 tsp]= 1 extra choice) .

Each serving:

2		Starch choices
1/2		Fats & Oils choice

MEXICAN CORN

500 ml	Frozen corn	2 cups
15 ml	Butter	1 tbsp
50 ml	Diced cooking onion	1/4 cup
50 ml	Diced green pepper	1/4 cup
50 ml	Diced red pepper	1/4 cup
2 ml	Salt	1/2 tsp
Pinch	Pepper	Pinch

☺ ☺ ☺ ☺ Makes 4 servings

1. In a microwave-safe dish, cover and microwave the corn on high until it is hot (4-5 minutes, depending on your microwave).
2. Meanwhile in a small saucepan, melt the butter over medium heat. Add the onions and peppers and cook until softened 2-3 minutes.
3. Stir the onions, peppers, salt and pepper into the hot corn and serve. Good with 'Soft Chicken Tacos' or burritos.

Did you know?

To steam vegetables in the microwave, cover the dish with plastic wrap (not wax paper) and do not add water as there is enough moisture on the vegetables to steam them. Be careful when you remove the plastic wrap because the steam is very hot even if the dish is not.

If you are not using the vegetables right away, plunging them into cold water will keep them a bright colour.

Each serving: (1/4 recipe)

1	■	Starch choice
1/2	▲	Fats & Oils choice
1	++	Extra choice

CARROT SALAD

500 ml	Grated carrot	2 cups
15 ml	Lemon juice	1 tbsp
15 ml	White wine vinegar	1 tbsp
15 ml	Vegetable oil	1 tbsp
5 ml	Splenda®	1 tsp
2 ml	Dijon mustard	1/2 tsp
Pinch	Salt & Pepper	Pinch
25 ml	Chopped fresh parsley	2 tbsp

☺ ☺ ☺ ☺ Makes 4 servings

1. Mix the peeled and grated carrots with the chopped parsley in a medium-sized glass bowl. Set aside.
2. In a small bowl, whisk together the lemon juice, vinegar, oil, Splenda®, mustard, salt and pepper.
3. Pour the dressing over the carrots and parsley and toss to coat. Cover and refrigerate for 1 hour or longer.

Did You Know?

If you are making dressing and you don't have a whisk, put the dressing ingredients in a jar with a tight fitting lid and shake.

Each serving: (1/4 recipe)

1	⬣	Fruit & Vegetable choice
1/2	▲	Fat choice

CAESAR SALAD

CAESAR DRESSING

175 ml	1% cottage cheese	3/4 cup
25 ml	Lemon juice	2 tbsp
7 ml	Dijon mustard	1 1/2 tsp
5 ml	Anchovy paste (optional)	1 tsp
5 ml	Worcestershire sauce	1 tsp
2	Cloves garlic, minced	2
2 ml each	Salt & Pepper	1/2 tsp each
10 ml	Olive oil	1 tsp
15 ml	'Light' sour cream	1 tbsp
50 ml	Parmesan cheese	1/4 cup

SALAD

1.5 L	Romaine lettuce	6 cups
50 ml	Parmesan Cheese	1/4 cup
375 ml	Croutons	1 1/2 cups

☺ ☺ ☺ ☺ ☺ ☺ Makes 6 servings

1. In a food processor, puree the cottage cheese and the lemon juice, Dijon, anchovy paste, Worcestershire sauce, garlic, salt and pepper. Add the olive oil and blend until thickened and smooth. Add the sour cream and parmesan cheese; blend. Refrigerate until serving time.

2. Wash romaine, pat dry with paper towels and tear into bite-size pieces.

3. Place lettuce in a large bowl. Pour dressing over lettuce and toss. Sprinkle with 50ml (1/4 cup) parmesan cheese and croutons, toss lightly and serve.

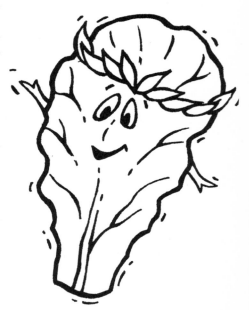

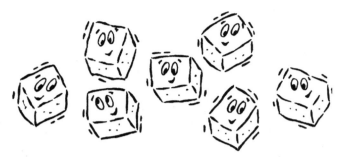

QUICK CROUTONS

Cut 2 slices of bread into small cubes. In a "Pyrex®" pie plate, toss together the cubed bread, 1 ml (1/4 tsp) of Italian herbs, 2 ml (1/2 tsp) of garlic powder, and 10 ml (2 tsp) of olive oil. Microwave on high for 3-4 minutes until crisp and golden, stopping and stirring once a minute.

Caesar salad must be eaten immediately after tossing or it gets limp. You can prepare the lettuce ahead and keep it crisp in a plastic bag with a paper towel in it, and you can prepare the dressing ahead and keep it in the refrigerator.

Each serving: (1/6 recipe)

1/2		Starch choice
1		Protein choice

1/2		Fats & Oils choice
1		Extra choice

CHICKEN SALAD NESTS

250 g	Cooked, diced chicken	1/2 lb
250 ml	Grapes, halved	1 cup
125 ml	Pineapple tidbits, drained	1/2 cup
50 ml	Diced celery	1/4 cup
25 ml	'No-fat' yogurt	2 tbsp
25 ml	'Light' mayonnaise	2 tbsp
2 ml	Salt	1/2 tsp
375 ml	Crisp chow mein noodles	1 1/2 cups
125 ml	Shredded carrot	1/2 cup
10 ml	Chopped chives or parsley	2 tsp

☺ ☺ ☺ ☺ Makes 4 servings

1. Combine the chicken, grapes, pineapple, celery, yogurt, mayonnaise, and salt in a mixing bowl. Cover and refrigerate for 1 hour to blend flavours.
2. Just before serving, combine noodles and carrots. Divide evenly onto 4 serving dishes; top with the chicken salad mixture and sprinkle with chopped chives or parsley.

Variation: Use chunk light tuna, packed in water, instead of chicken.

250 ml (1 cup) of pineapple packed in syrup has one sugars choice more than pineapple packed in its own juice. Always use canned fruit that is packed in its own juice or in pear juice.

Each serving: (1/4 recipe)

1	■ Starch choices		2	⬤ Protein choices	
1	⬢ Fruit & Vegetable choice		1	▲ Fats & Oils choice	

CHICKEN FAJITA SALAD

500 grams	4 Skinned, boned chicken breasts	1 lb
10 ml	Vegetable oil	2 tsp
25 ml	Lime juice	2 tbsp
15 ml	Splenda®	1 tbsp
10 ml	Chili powder	2 tsp
2	Cloves garlic, minced	2
1 L	Shredded lettuce	4 cups
2	Tomatoes, diced	2
1	Avocado, diced	1
3	Green onions, sliced	3
	Pitted black olives, optional	
6 - 22 cm	Flour tortillas	6 - 8"

☺ ☺ ☺ ☺ ☺ ☺ Makes 6 servings

1. In a medium-sized non-metal bowl, combine the vegetable oil, lime juice, Splenda®, chili powder, and garlic. Add the chicken, turning it to coat both sides. Cover and refrigerate for 1 to 2 hours.
2. Make tortilla shells (instructions below) and set aside.
3. Preheat the broiler with the rack 15cm (6") from the element. Line the broiler pan with foil.
4. Broil the chicken 8 minutes, turn, brush with marinade and broil the other side for 7-8 minutes or until it is tender and the juices run clear.
5. While the chicken is cooking, prepare the salad ingredients.
6. To serve: cut the chicken into strips. Divide the lettuce evenly into each tortilla shell. Top with the chicken, tomato, avocado, green onions, and olives. Serve with salsa if desired.

TORTILLA SHELLS

Preheat oven to 200° (400°F). Invert 6 custard cups on 2 cookie sheets; spray with vegetable oil spray. Place one tortilla over each cup (tortillas will mold to cups while baking). Spray tortillas with vegetable oil spray. Bake at 200° (400°F) for 6-7 minutes or until crisp and golden. Remove from custard cups and cool.

Each serving: (1 filled tortilla shell)

1	■	Starch choice	2 1/2	◒	Protein choices
1/2	◆	Fruit & Vegetable choice	1/2	▲	Fats & Oils choice

FAVOURITE FRUIT SALAD

500 ml	Cubed watermelon	2 cups
250 ml	Seedless grapes	1 cup
250 ml	Miniature marshmallows	1 cup
250 ml	Mandarin orange (in light syrup)	1 cup
250 ml	Pineapple tidbits (canned in juice)	1 cup

☺ ☺ ☺ ☺ ☺ ☺ ☺ ☺ Makes 8 servings

1.   Drain the canned mandarin oranges and the pineapple tidbits well.
2.   Combine all the ingredients in a medium sized bowl. Toss gently.
3.   Refrigerate until serving time.

Each serving: (1/8 recipe)

1 1/2   Fruit & Vegetable choices

1/2   Sugar choice

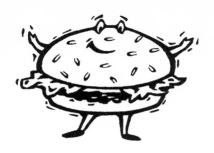

BURGERS, SANDWICHES & PIZZAS

Page		Carbohydrates	Proteins	Fats	Calories	Kilojoules
60	**Adam's Meatball Subs**	39	20	12	337	1415
62	**Open-face Deli Melts**	27	23	6	261	1096
63	**Tuna Melt On Pita**	32	27	9	321	1348
64	**Picnic Hero**	40	23	8	336	1411
65	**Salad Bar Sub (Egg Salad)**	36	14	13	317	1331
65	**Salad Bar Sub (Tuna Salad)**	35	24	8	317	1331
67	**Turkey Burger Melts**	33	25	12	345	1449
68	**Teriyaki Burgers**	36	28	11	380	1596
69	**Chili Burgers**	38	33	30	562	2360
70	**Fillet Of Fish Burgers**	38	20	4	273	1147
71	**Light Tartar Sauce**	2	1	3	38	160
72	**Tuna Burgers**	32	27	14	368	1546
73	**French Bread Pizza**	43	29	27	537	2255
75	**Easy Pizza Dough**	37	6	1	175	735
76	**Sloppy Joe Pizza**	42	21	11	352	1478
77	**Taco Pizza**	39	22	9	322	1352
78	**Funny Face Pizza**	41	16	12	334	1403
79	**Virtuous Veggie Pizza**	47	20	8	334	1403
80	**Hot Dog Kabobs**	39	10	15	326	1369

Nutritional Analysis (per Serving)

ADAM'S MEATBALL SUBS

BARBECUE SAUCE

5 ml	Vegetable oil	1 tsp
50 ml	Chopped onion	1/4 cup
50 ml	Chopped green pepper	1/4 cup
1	Can (213 g/7.5 oz) tomato sauce	1
45 ml	Ketchup	3 tbsp
45 ml	Splenda®	3 tbsp
25 ml	Red wine vinegar	2 tbsp
2 ml	Worcestershire sauce	1/2 tsp
2 ml	Salt	1/2 tsp

MEATBALLS

500 g	Lean ground beef	1 lb
25 ml	Dry bread crumbs	2 tbsp
25 ml	Minced onion	2 tbsp
2 ml	Salt	1/2 tsp
1 ml	Pepper	1/4 tsp
1 ml	Garlic powder	1/4 tsp
2 ml	Worcestershire sauce	1/2 tsp
1	Egg white	1
6	Small sub or hero buns	6

☺ ☺ ☺ ☺ ☺ ☺ Makes 6 servings

BARBECUE SAUCE

1. Heat the vegetable oil in a medium-sized saucepan. Add 50 ml (1/4 cup) chopped onion and green pepper, sauté just until tender (about 2 minutes).
2. Add the tomato sauce, ketchup, Splenda®, vinegar, 2 ml (1/2tsp) Worcestershire sauce and 2 ml (1/2 tsp) of salt. Simmer, uncovered, for 15 minutes

ADAM'S MEATBALL SUBS CONTINUED

MEATBALLS

1. In a medium-sized mixing bowl, combine the ground beef, bread crumbs, onion, 2 ml (1/2 tsp) salt, 1 ml (1/4 tsp) pepper, garlic powder, 2 ml (1/2 tsp) Worcestershire sauce, and the egg white. Mix well.
2. Using a heaping teaspoon for each, shape into 20 meatballs.
3. Spray a large skillet with vegetable oil spray and fry the meatballs until brown on all sides and cooked through.

To serve:

1. Cut the buns in half and put 4 meatballs on each bun.
2. Spoon the hot barbecue sauce over the meatballs, replace the top half of the bun and serve.

Did you know?

When cooking lean ground meats, adding egg whites and bread crumbs helps bind the meat together so that it won't crumble while cooking.

Each serving: (1 sandwich)

2		Starch choices	2		Protein choices
1		Fruit & Vegetable choice	1	▲	Fats & Oils choice

OPEN-FACE DELI MELTS

1	Medium onion, sliced	1
1	Green pepper, sliced	1
25 ml	'Fat-free' Ranch dressing	2 tbsp
2	Bagels (split)	2
	Dijon mustard	
250 g	Sliced turkey, ham or lean beef	1/2 lb
125 ml	Grated Swiss cheese	1/2 cup

☺ ☺ ☺ ☺ Makes 4 servings

1. Place the sliced onions and peppers in a microwave-safe baking dish, cover (with a non-metallic lid or plastic wrap) and cook for 4 to 5 minutes. Stir halfway through cooking.
2. Drain and then toss with the ranch dressing.
3. Spread the bagel halves with mustard; top with meat and then sprinkle with cheese.
4. Place on a baking sheet and broil until the cheese is melted.
5. Top each sandwich with some of the onion mixture and serve.

Did You Know?

You can use your favourite lean deli meat. Roast beef, corned beef, ham and turkey are almost identical in terms of fat content.

Each serving: (1/2 bagel)

1 1/2	■	Starch choices
1/2		Fruit & Vegetable choice
2 1/2		Protein choices

TUNA MELT ON PITA

50 m	'Light' mayonnaise	1/4 cup
6	15 cm (6") Pita breads	6
2	Cans (213 g/7.5 oz) flaked water-packed tuna, drained	2
50 ml	Chopped celery	1/4 cup
50 ml	Minced green onion	1/4 cup
2	Chopped dill pickles	2
250 ml	Grated 'light' cheddar cheese	1 cup

☺ ☺ ☺ ☺ ☺ ☺ Makes 6 servings

1. Preheat the broiler with the oven rack 10cm (4–5") from the element.
2. Spread 5ml (1 tsp) of mayonnaise on each pita.
3. Combine the tuna, celery, green onions, pickles and remaining mayonnaise in a small mixing bowl.
4. Spread the tuna mixture over the pitas and sprinkle evenly with the grated cheese.
5. Place on a cookie sheet and broil for 3 minutes or until hot and bubbling.

Did You Know?

Always choose water-packed tuna. A 85g (3 oz) serving of water-packed tuna only has 1 gram of fat while the same amount of oil-packed tuna has 8 to 12 grams of fat.

Each serving: (1 pita)

2	■	Starch choices
3	⊘	Protein choices
1	++	Extra choice

PICNIC HERO

1	Loaf (375 g/12oz)French bread	1
	Mustard/cream cheese spread	
2	Dill pickles, thinly sliced	2
12	Lettuce leaves	12
284 g	Thinly sliced turkey	10 oz
4 slices	'Light' processed Swiss cheese	4 slices
1	Large tomato, thinly sliced	1
1/2	Red onion, thinly sliced (optional)	1/2
250 ml	Alfalfa sprouts	1 cup
45 ml	'Light' mayonnaise	3 tbsp

MUSTARD/CREAM CHEESE SPREAD:

45 ml	'Light' soft cream cheese	3 tbsp
10 ml	Dijon mustard	2 tsp
15 ml	'Light' sour cream	1 tbsp
2 ml	Horseradish	1/2 tsp

☺ ☺ ☺ ☺ ☺ ☺ Makes 6 servings

1. In a small bowl, combine the 'mustard/cream cheese spread' ingredients.
2. Cut the bread in half lengthways and spread the bottom half with the mustard/cream cheese spread.
3. Layer the pickles, lettuce, and turkey on the cheese spread.
4. Cut the Swiss cheese in half diagonally and arrange it on top of the turkey.
5. Continue to layer with the tomatoes, onions and sprouts.
6. Spread the top half of the bread with the mayonnaise and place it on the top.
7. Cut into 6 slices to serve or wrap well and slice just before serving.

Each serving: (1/6 recipe)

2 1/2		Starch choices
2 1/2		Protein choices
1		Extra choice

SALAD BAR SUBS

In a medium sized bowl, mix the salad filling of your choice:

LIGHT EGG SALAD:

4	Eggs, hard boiled	4
1/4	Green pepper, diced	1/4
2	Small green onions, sliced	2
25 ml	'Light' mayonnaise	2 tbsp
5 ml	Dijon mustard (optional)	1 tsp

☺ ☺ ☺ ☺ Makes 4 servings

To make the egg salad filling:

1. Chop 2 whole eggs and 2 egg whites (discard the remaining 2 yolks).
2. Combine with the diced green pepper, the sliced green onions, 25 ml (2 tbsp) of mayonnaise and 5 ml (1 tsp) of Dijon. Season with salt and pepper to taste.

TUNA EGG SALAD:

1	Can (213g/7.5 oz) tuna (packed in water)	1
2	Hard-cooked egg whites	2
25 ml	Grated carrot	2 tbsp
2	Small green onions, sliced	2
25 ml	'Light' mayonnaise	2 tbsp

☺ ☺ ☺ ☺ Makes 4 servings

To make the tuna salad filling:

1. Drain the tuna and flake with a fork in a medium-sized mixing bowl.
2. Chop the egg white and stir into the tuna along with the grated carrot, the green onions, and 25 ml (2 tbsp) of mayonnaise.

Continued next page…

SALAD BAR SUBS CONTINUED...

SUBMARINE SANDWICH:

4	Small submarine buns (or Kaisers)	4
25 ml	'Light' mayonnaise	2 tbsp
8	Lettuce leaves	8
1	Large tomato, thinly sliced	1
1/2	Cucumber, thinly sliced	1/2
250 ml	Alfalfa sprouts	1 cup
4	Slices bacon, cooked	4

☺ ☺ ☺ ☺ Makes 4 servings

To make the subs:

1. Slice each bun in half. Spread both sides with 'light' mayonnaise.
2. Arrange the lettuce on the bottom half of the buns.
3. Dividing the ingredients between the four buns, spoon on the egg OR tuna salad and then top with the tomato, cucumber, alfalfa sprouts, bacon and the bun top.

Each serving: **WITH EGG SALAD**   Each serving: **WITH TUNA SALAD**

2	■	Starch choices		2	■	Starch choices
1/2	◆	Fruit & Vegetable		1/2	◆	Fruit & Vegetable
1 1/2	⬤	Protein choices		3	⬤	Protein choices
1 1/2	▲	Fats & Oils choices				

TURKEY BURGER MELTS

1	Egg white	1
50 ml	Minced green onions (optional)	1/4 cup
50 ml	Minced parsley (optional)	1/4 cup
25 ml	Bread or cracker crumbs	2 tbsp
25 ml	Water	2 tbsp
5 ml	Dijon mustard	1 tsp
2 ml each	Salt, garlic, basil	1/2 tsp each
500 g	Ground turkey (or chicken)	1 lb
250 ml	Grated part skim mozzarella	1 cup
6	Hamburger or Kaiser buns	6

Optional toppings: Tomatoes, lettuce, pickles, fried onions and mushrooms.

☺ ☺ ☺ ☺ ☺ ☺ Makes 6 servings

1. In a medium-sized mixing bowl, mix together the egg white, onions, parsley, bread crumbs, water, mustard, salt, garlic and basil. Mix in the ground turkey. Use hands to mix thoroughly.
2. Shape into 6 patties.
3. Barbecue about 7 minutes per side or fry in a lightly greased non-stick skillet.
4. Top with cheese and cook until the cheese melts.
5. Serve on fresh Kaiser buns or in hamburger pitas stuffed with fresh lettuce and sliced pickles. (Don't forget to count the fats & oils choice if you add mayonnaise!)

CAUTION!

Be sure to thoroughly wash your hands and preparation area with lots of soap after touching raw poultry.

Each serving:

2	■	Starch choices	1/2	▲	Fats & Oils choice
3		Protein choices	1	++	Extra choice

TERIYAKI BURGERS

500 g	Extra lean ground beef	1 lb
250 ml	Chopped water chestnuts	1 cup
1	Egg white	1
25 ml	Bread crumbs	2 tbsp

MARINADE:

25 ml	Sliced green onions	2 tbsp
25 ml	Splenda®	2 tbsp
2 ml	Grated ginger root	1/2 tsp
1	Clove garlic, minced	1
50 ml	Soy sauce (low sodium)	1/4 cup
4	Crusty hamburger buns	4

Optional topping (2 slices = 1 fruit & vegetable choice)
Sliced pineapple (in its own juice)

☺ ☺ ☺ ☺ Makes 4 servings

1. In a medium-sized bowl, combine the ground beef, chopped water chestnuts, egg white and bread crumbs. Shape into 4 patties.
2. Place patties in a glass baking dish.
3. In a small bowl, combine marinade ingredients. Pour over the hamburger patties. Cover and refrigerate for one hour or more.
4. Barbecue for 7 minutes, turn, brush with marinade and barbecue for 7–8 minutes or until done.
5. Top each with 2 pineapple slices, if desired, and serve on buns.

Did You Know?

As a general rule, 120g (4 oz) of raw meat will yield 90g (3 oz) when cooked.

Each serving:

2 1/2		Starch choices
3		Protein choices
1/2		Fats & Oils choice

CHILI BURGERS

125 ml	Chopped onion	1/2 cup
50 ml	Chopped green pepper	1/4 cup
1	Clove garlic, minced	1
5 ml	Vegetable oil	1 tsp
375 ml	Canned chili with beans	1 1/2 cups
500 g	Lean ground beef	1 lb
6	Hamburger buns	6
250 ml	Grated 'light' cheddar cheese	1 cup

Optional toppings:
Shredded lettuce, green pepper, and onion slices

☺ ☺ ☺ ☺ ☺ ☺ Makes 6 servings

1. Measure the vegetable oil into a medium-sized saucepan. Add the onions, green pepper and garlic, cooking until softened (about 2 minutes). Add the chili and simmer while preparing the burgers.
2. Shape the hamburger into 6 patties. Grill on the barbecue (about 7 minutes per side or until cooked through).
3. Toast the hamburger buns, if desired.
4. To assemble the chili burgers, place the shredded lettuce on the bottom half of the bun, top with a hamburger patty, 50 ml (1/4 cup) of the chili, 45 ml (3 tbsp) of the grated cheese, the pepper and onion slices, more lettuce and then the top half of the bun.

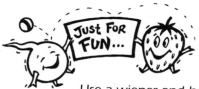

Use a wiener and hot dog bun to make a chili cheese dog!

Each serving:

2	■	Starch choices
4	⊘	Protein choices
3 1/2	▲	Fats & Oils choices

FILLET OF FISH BURGERS

500 g	White fish fillets, eg., cod or sole	1 lb
125 ml	Cornflake crumbs	1/2 cup
50 ml	Parmesan cheese	1/4 cup
2	Egg whites	2
15 ml	Vegetable oil	1 tbsp
6	Whole wheat crusty buns or Hamburger pita halves	6

Optional toppings:
Lettuce, dill pickles, tomato and onion slices, 'light tartar sauce'

☺ ☺ ☺ ☺ ☺ ☺ Makes 6 servings

1. Cut the fish fillets into six equal pieces.
2. Preheat the oven to 220° (425°F). Spray a baking pan with vegetable oil spray.
3. In a shallow dish or pie plate, beat the egg and oil together with a fork.
4. In a separate shallow dish, combine the parmesan cheese and the corn flake crumbs. Dip the fish pieces into the egg mixture and then into the crumbs. Press the crumbs on to stick.
5. Place the fish on the baking pan and bake for 18–20 minutes or until the fish flakes easily when tested with a fork. Don't overcook.
6. Serve on whole wheat rolls or in pitas. Top with 15 ml (1 tbsp) 'light tartar sauce', add lettuce, tomatoes, onions and pickles, as desired.

Did You Know?

White fish fillets are very similar in terms of taste and nutrition, so choose what you like and what is available when cooking with fish.

Each serving:

2 1/2		Starch choices
2	⊘	Protein choices

LIGHT
TARTAR SAUCE

125 ml	'No-fat' yogurt	1/2 cup
75 ml	'Light' mayonnaise	1/3 cup
25 ml	Chopped dill pickles	2 tbsp
5 ml	Lemon juice	1 tsp
2 ml	Dijon mustard	1/2 tsp
	Dash of tabasco and	
	Worcestershire Sauce	

☺ ☺ ☺ ☺ ☺ ☺ Makes 6 servings

1.   Stir all the ingredients together in a small bowl. Chill. Serve with fish or on fish burgers.

Each serving: (25 ml (2 tbsp))   or   Each serving: (15 ml (1 tbsp))

| 1/2 | ▲ | Fat choice | 1 | ++ | Extra choice |

| 1 | ++ | Extra choice |

TUNA BURGERS

250 ml	Grated 'light' cheddar cheese	1 cup
1	Hard-cooked egg, chopped	1
1	Hard-cooked egg white	1
1	Can (213g/7.5oz) water-packed tuna, drained	1
15 ml	Minced green onion	1 tbsp
15 ml	Minced green pepper	1 tbsp
15 ml	Minced dill pickle	1 tbsp
50 ml	'Light' mayonnaise	1/4 cup
4	Hamburger buns	4

☺ ☺ ☺ ☺ Makes 4 servings

1. Chop the hard-boiled egg and egg white. Mince the green onions, green peppers, and pickles. Drain the tuna fish and flake it with a fork. Cut the buns in half.
2. Mix the grated cheese, chopped eggs, tuna, onions, peppers, pickles, and mayonnaise in a small bowl.
3. Divide the mixture into four equal portions and spread it on the bun bottoms. Replace the tops of the buns and wrap each bun individually in foil.
4. Grill the burger packages on the barbecue for 20 minutes or bake them in the oven at 180° (350°F).
5. Unwrap carefully and serve.

Did You Know?

To hard-cook eggs; place the eggs in a saucepan and cover them with cold water. Heat to boiling; reduce heat and simmer for 15 minutes. Cool the eggs under cold water to stop cooking.

Each serving:

| 2 | | Starch choices | 1 | ▲ | Fats & Oils choice |
| 3 | ⊘ | Protein choices | 1 |  | Extra choice |

FRENCH BREAD PIZZA

1	Small (250g/8oz) loaf French bread	1
125 ml	Pizza or spaghetti sauce	1/2 cup
500 ml	Grated part skim mozzarella cheese	2 cups
125 g	Chopped pepperoni	4 oz

Topping options (125 ml [1/2 cup] = 1 extra choice):

2	Green onions, sliced	2
500 ml	Sliced mushrooms	2 cups
125 ml	Chopped green pepper	1/2 cup
1	Tomato, diced	1

☺ ☺ ☺ ☺ Makes 4 servings

1. Cut the French bread in half lengthways and toast lightly 10–15 cm (4–6") under the broiler, cut side up.
2. Prepare your selection of the toppings: slice the green onions, slice and micro-cook the mushrooms (for 2 minutes or until soft), dice the peppers and tomatoes.
3. Mix the toppings in a medium-sized bowl. Add the pepperoni and cheese, toss lightly to mix.
4. Spread the pizza sauce on the toasted bread; spoon on the topping.
5. Cook under the broiler for 3–4 minutes, until the cheese is melted.
6. Cut into 4 pieces to serve.

Variations continued next page

Each serving: (1/4 recipe)

2 1/2	Starch choices	3 1/2 Protein choices
1/2	Fruit & vegetable choice	3 1/2 Fats & Oils choices

FRENCH BREAD PIZZA
VARIATIONS

---

1. **CHICKEN FAJITA PIZZA BREAD**

   Use salsa instead of pizza sauce, and cooked slivered chicken instead of pepperoni, omit mushrooms, add red peppers and use Monterey Jack cheese instead of mozzarella.

2. **GREEK PIZZA BREAD**

   Omit pepperoni and mushrooms. Add sliced black olives, and 250g (1/2 lb) shrimp. Substitute 150 ml (2/3 cup) crumbled feta for 150 ml (2/3 cup) of the mozzarella.

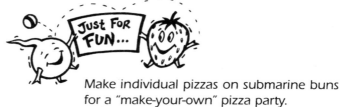

Make individual pizzas on submarine buns for a "make-your-own" pizza party.

EASY PIZZA DOUGH

Easy pizza dough:

375 ml	All-purpose flour	1 1/2 cups
175 ml	Whole wheat flour	3/4 cup
1	Envelope rapid-rise yeast	1
5 ml	Salt	1 tsp
2 ml	Granulated sugar	1/2 tsp
175 ml	Hot tap water	3/4 cup

☺ ☺ ☺ ☺ ☺ ☺ Makes 6 servings

1. Stir together the flours, yeast, salt and sugar either in a food processor or in a large bowl with a wooden spoon. Add the water and stir until the dough forms a ball (if you need to use more water, add 15 ml (1 tbsp) at a time). Process for one minute or knead for 3 or 4 minutes by hand.
2. Cover the dough with plastic wrap and let it rise for 10 minutes.
3. Divide the dough into 6 pieces for individual pizzas or leave it in one ball for a large pizza.
4. Sprinkle a baking sheet or pizza pan lightly with cornmeal and then with lightly buttered fingers, spread the dough into round pizza shapes.
5. Top with one of the following 'Four Way' suggested toppings.

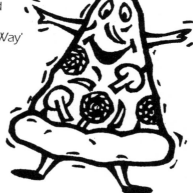

Each serving: (1/6 recipe)

2   Starch choices

SLOPPY JOE PIZZA

250 g	Lean ground beef	1/2 lb
125 ml	Chopped onion	1/2 cup
1	Clove garlic, minced	1
175 ml	Spaghetti sauce	3/4 cup
2 ml	Chili powder	1/2 tsp
375 ml	Shredded part skim mozzarella cheese	1 1/2 cups

☺ ☺ ☺ ☺ ☺ ☺ Makes 6 servings

1. In a large skillet, cook the lean ground beef over medium heat for 3 minutes, stirring occasionally.
2. Add the onions and garlic; cook until the meat is brown and crumbly and the onion is tender.
3. Stir in the spaghetti sauce, the chili powder and a dash of salt and pepper.
4. Spread the meat sauce onto the pizza shells; sprinkle the cheese over top.
5. Bake in a 200° (400°F) over for 15 minutes.

Each serving: (1/6 recipe)

2	■ Starch choices	2	⊘ Protein choices
1	◢ Fruit & vegetable choice	1	▲ Fats & Oils choice

FOUR WAYS TOPPING
TACO PIZZA

250 g	Lean ground turkey	1/2 lb
125 ml	Chopped onion	1/2 cup
1/2	Package taco seasoning mix	1/2
375 ml	Shredded part skim mozzarella cheese	1 1/2 cup
	Your favourite taco toppings	

☺ ☺ ☺ ☺ ☺ ☺ Makes 6 servings

1. In a large skillet, cook the ground turkey over medium heat for 3 minutes, stirring occasionally so that it is crumbly.
2. Add the onions and cook until the meat is brown.
3. Add the taco seasoning and 50 ml (1/4 cup) of water. Simmer for 10 minutes.
4. Spread the taco meat on the pizza shells; sprinkle the cheese over top.
5. Bake in a 200° (400°F) over for 15 minutes.
6. Serve topped with your favourite taco toppings; chopped tomato, chopped onions, lettuce, salsa, and 'no-fat' sour cream.

Each serving: (1/6 recipe)

2		Starch choices
1/2		Fruit & vegetable choice
2 1/2		Protein choices

FOUR WAYS TOPPING
FUNNY FACE PIZZA

500 ml	Pizza or spaghetti sauce	2 cups
500 ml	Grated part skim mozzarella cheese	2 cups
60 g	Pepperoni (12 slices)	3 1/2 oz
	Selection of green pepper slices, black olives, and grated carrots	

☺ ☺ ☺ ☺ ☺ ☺ ☺ ☺ Makes 8 servings

1.	Divide the pizza dough into 8 balls (instead of six), and spread 8 shells on a baking sheet.
2.	Spread the shells with the spaghetti sauce and then sprinkle with the cheese.
3.	Arrange the toppings on the cheese to look like funny faces.
4.	Bake at 200° (400°F) for 15 minutes. Garnish each pizza with grated carrots for hair.

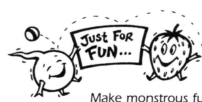

Make monstrous funny face pizzas for Halloween.

Each serving: (1/8 recipe)

| 2 | | Starch choices | 1 1/2 | | Protein choices |
| 1 | | Fruit & vegetable choice | 1 1/2 | | Fats & Oils choices |

FOUR WAYS TOPPING
VIRTUOUS VEGGIE PIZZA

1	Can (398ml/14 oz) Italian stewed tomatoes	1
500 ml	Grated part skim mozzarella cheese	2 cups
500 ml	Broccoli florets	2 cups
250 ml	Sliced carrots and/or zucchini	1 cup
250 ml	Sliced mushrooms	1 cup
1	Red or green pepper, chopped	1
25 ml	Parmesan cheese	2 tbsp

☺ ☺ ☺ ☺ ☺ ☺ Makes 6 servings

1. Cook the vegetables until tender-crisp in the microwave (2–3 minutes), then rinse under cold water and drain.
2. Sprinkle half of the mozzarella onto the pizza shells. Spoon the tomatoes onto the mozzarella, then top with the vegetables.
3. Sprinkle the remaining mozzarella and the parmesan over all.
4. Bake at 200° (400°F) for 15 minutes.

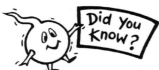

To cook your vegetables perfectly you can:

a) Cook them separately in the microwave (some cook faster than others). Cover a microwave-safe bowl with plastic wrap and then cook on high 2–4 minutes, checking and stirring after 2 minutes, or

b) cook in a saucepan of boiling water for 3–5 minutes, drain and immediately rinse with cold water to keep the colours bright.

Each serving: (1/6 recipe)

2		Starch choices	2		Protein choices
1 1/2		Fruit & vegetable choices	1/2		Fats & Oils choice

HOT DOG KABOBS

4	All-beef wieners	4
4	Hot dog buns	4
4	Cherry tomatoes	4
50 ml	Green pepper chunks	1/4 cup
125 ml	Pineapple chunks	1/2 cup
50 ml	Barbeque sauce	1/4 cup

☺ ☺ ☺ ☺ Makes 4 servings

1. Cut wieners into 5 pieces each. Thread the wiener pieces onto skewers alternating with green pepper pieces, and pineapple chunks. Top each skewer with a cherry tomato.
2. Brush lightly with barbeque sauce.
3. Grill over hot coals until lightly browned.
4. Serve on toasted hot dog buns.
5. Serve with dill pickles, chopped onion, mustard, or ketchup.

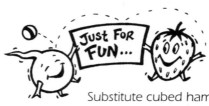

Substitute cubed ham or cooked sausage for the wieners.

Each serving: (1 sandwich)

| 2 | | Starch choices | 1 | | Protein choice |
| 1/2 | | Fruit & vegetable choice | 2 1/2 | | Fats & Oils choices |

DINNERS

Page		Carbohydrates	Proteins	Fats	Calories	Kilojoules
82	**Crunchy Peanut Fish Fillets**	15	23	11	254	1067
83	**Fish Sticks**	15	19	2	160	672
84	**Salmon Croquettes**	5	13	6	130	546
85	**Soft Chicken Tacos**	33	32	11	375	1575
86	**Orange Glazed Chicken Wings**	15	18	14	249	1046
87	**Chicken Fingers**	12	22	5	190	798
87	**Plum Sauce**	4	0	0	14	59
88	**Oven-baked Crispy Chicken**	16	29	7	245	1029
89	**Tex's Tacos**	35	26	20	428	1798
90	**Garden Burritos**	32	12	8	238	1000
91	**Chili Con Carne**	26	24	11	299	1256
92	**Refrito Burritos**	30	15	7	235	987
93	**Hawaiian Chili**	48	20	6	320	1344
94	**Salmon & Cheddar Macaroni**	37	24	14	365	1546
95	**Lasagna (For 6)**	35	37	14	405	1701
95	**Lasagna (For 8)**	26	28	10	303	1273
97	**Lasagna Roll-ups**	39	23	10	337	1415
98	**Spaghetti & Meatball Skillet**	21	25	15	320	1344
99	**Sweet & Sour Meatballs**	68	30	20	560	2352
100	**Fettuccini Alfredo (Egg noodles)**	32	12	7	237	995

Nutritional Analysis (per Serving)

CRUNCHY PEANUT FISH FILLETS

250 ml	Bread crumbs	1 cup
50 ml	Chopped dry-roasted peanuts	1/4 cup
2 ml	Salt	1/2 tsp
2 ml	Pepper	1/2 tsp
2	Eggs	2
15 ml	Vegetable oil	1 tbsp
500 g	Fish fillets	1 lb
	(sole, cod or other white fish)	

☺ ☺ ☺ ☺ ☺ Makes 5 servings

1. Preheat the oven to 220° (425°F). Spray a baking sheet with vegetable oil spray.
2. Combine the bread crumbs, peanuts, salt and pepper in a food processor and process until finely chopped. Pour into a shallow dish (such as a pie plate).
3. Beat the eggs and vegetable oil together in a small bowl, with a fork.
4. Dip each fish fillet into the egg mixture and then into the crumbs. Place on the baking sheet.
5. Bake at 220° (425°F) for 6 minutes. Turn and bake for 5 minutes more. Test for doneness.

Did You Know?

Upon heating, fish will turn from translucent to opaque. Fish is cooked when it is opaque throughout and flakes easily when pierced with a fork.

Each serving: (1/5 recipe)

1	■	Starch choice
3	⊘	Protein choices
1/2	▲	Fats & Oils choice

FISH STICKS

375 g	Firm white fish (eg. cod or halibut)	3/4 lb
250 ml	Whole wheat bread crumbs	1 cup
25 ml	'Light' mayonnaise	2 tbsp
2 ml	Salt	1/2 tsp
1 ml	Pepper	1/4 tsp
Pinch	Thyme	Pinch
1	Egg white	1

☺ ☺ ☺ ☺ Makes 4 servings

1. Preheat the oven to 220° (425°F). Spray a baking sheet lightly with vegetable oil spray.
2. Cut the fish crosswise into 8 sticks.
3. In a small shallow bowl, combine the bread crumbs, mayonnaise, salt, pepper and thyme.
4. In a separate bowl, beat the egg white with a fork.
5. Dip the fish sticks in the egg white and then roll them in the crumbs, pressing the crumbs on with your fingers.
6. Arrange the fish sticks on the baking sheet and sprinkle with any remaining crumbs.
7. Bake at 220° (425°F) for 15 minutes. Serve with 'light tartar sauce' or ketchup.

Eggs are good sources of proteins, vitamins and minerals. The egg yolks contain fat that the egg whites do not. A simple way to reduce fat is to use egg whites instead of the whole eggs.

Each serving: (2 fish sticks)

1	■	Starch choice
2		Protein choices

SALMON CROQUETTES

1	Can (213g/7.5oz) sockeye salmon	1
1	Egg	1
50 ml	Bread crumbs	1/4 cup
1 ml	Lemon juice	1/4 tsp
25 ml	Grated onion	2 tbsp
10 ml	'Light' mayonnaise	2 tsp
dash	Salt & pepper	dash
10 ml	Vegetable oil	2 tsp

☺ ☺ ☺ ☺ Makes 4 servings

1. Drain the salmon and place in a medium-sized mixing bowl. Remove the bones, mash with a fork.
2. Add all of the remaining ingredients, except the vegetable oil.
3. Form into 8 small patties and refrigerate for 30 minutes or more.
4. Heat the oil in a large non-stick skillet. Fry the patties over medium heat, turning them only once, until golden. (About 8–10 minutes per side.)
5. Serve hot with 'light tartar sauce'.

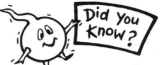

Use your imagination to make meals fun. For Valentine's Day try making heart-shaped Salmon Croquettes and pink Fettuccini Alfredo (add pink food colouring to the sauce).

Each serving: (2 croquettes)

1/2		Fruit & vegetable choice
2	⊘	Protein choices

SOFT CHICKEN TACOS

3	Boneless chicken breasts	3
8 - 22 cm	Flour tortillas	8 - 8"
1	Cooking onion, diced	1
1/2 pkg	Taco seasoning mix	1/2 pkg
125 ml	Salsa	1/2 cup
250 ml	Grated Monterey Jack cheese	1 cup

Optional toppings:

1/2	Green pepper, chopped	1/2
1	Tomato, chopped	1
250 ml	Shredded lettuce	1 cup
125 ml	0.1% sour cream	1/2 cup

☺ ☺ ☺ ☺ Makes 4 servings

1. Preheat the oven to 180° (350°F).
2. Remove the skin and fat from the chicken. Cut into thin strips. Stir-fry the chicken strips in 5ml (1 tsp) of vegetable oil in a large skillet until no longer pink (about 5 minutes). Add the diced onion to the pan and stir-fry for 1 minute. Add the taco seasoning and 125 ml (1/2 cup) water to the chicken and onion, simmer for 10 minutes.
3. Meanwhile, wrap the tortillas in foil. Place in the oven for 10 minutes.
4. Prepare optional toppings and place in small serving bowls.
5. Remove the tortillas from the oven and unwrap, being careful of steam.
6. To serve: spoon the chicken onto the hot tortillas, top with grated cheese, salsa, and optional toppings. Fold tortillas in half and eat with a knife and fork. (125 ml [1/2 c] optional vegetable = 1 extra choice)

Each serving: (2 tacos)

2	■	Starch choices
4	⊘	Protein choices
1	++	Extra choice

ORANGE GLAZED CHICKEN WINGS

12	Chicken wings	12
50 ml	Frozen orange juice concentrate	1/4 cup
25 ml	Honey	2 tbsp
25 ml	Splenda®	2 tbsp
50 ml	Soy sauce (low sodium)	1/4 cup
2 ml	Ground ginger	1/2 tsp
2 ml	Garlic powder	1/2 tsp
2 ml	Salt	1/2 tsp

☺ ☺ ☺ ☺ ☺ ☺ Makes 6 servings

1. Place the chicken wings in a plastic or glass bowl.
2. Combine the orange juice concentrate, honey, Splenda®, soy sauce, ginger, salt and garlic in a small bowl. Mix well. Pour over the wings.
3. Let the wings marinate for at least one hour in the refrigerator.
4. Preheat oven to 190° (375°F).
5. Remove the wings from the marinade and arrange them on a foil-lined baking sheet.
6. Pour the remaining marinade into a small saucepan and bring to a boil. Remove from heat.
7. Meanwhile bake the wings for 20 minutes, turn. Brush with the reserved marinade and continue baking for another 20 minutes.

Always rinse raw chicken and pat it dry with paper towels before cooking to remove any surface bacteria.

Each serving: (2 wings)

1/2		Fruit & Vegetable choice	2 1/2	◓	Protein choices
1	✳	Sugars choice	1 1/2	▲	Fats & Oils choices

CHICKEN FINGERS WITH PLUM SAUCE

4 (454g)	Boneless chicken breasts	4 (1 lb)
24	Soda crackers	24
50 ml	'Light' mayonnaise	1/4 cup

PLUM DIPPING SAUCE

25 ml	Plum sauce	2 tbsp
15 ml	Ketchup	1 tbsp
15 ml	Soy sauce (low sodium)	1 tbsp
5 ml	Vinegar	1 tsp
5 ml	Splenda®	1 tsp

☺ ☺ ☺ ☺ ☺ Makes 5 servings

1. Preheat the oven to 200° (400°F). Spray a baking sheet with vegetable oil spray.
2. Crush the crackers in a food processor or place the crackers in a plastic bag and crush with a rolling pin. Pour into a shallow dish.
3. Spoon the mayonnaise into a separate dish.
4. Rinse the chicken, pat dry with paper towels, and remove the skin. Using a sharp knife, cut each breast into 6 strips.
5. Add the chicken to the mayonnaise and mix to coat each strip. Roll the coated chicken strips, one at a time, in cracker crumbs and arrange in a single layer on the prepared baking sheet.
6. Bake for 15 minutes, turn the strips, and bake for 10 to 15 minutes longer (until golden and crisp).
7. Meanwhile, combine all the plum dipping sauce ingredients in a small bowl and serve with the chicken strips.

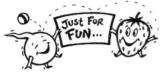

You can use crushed Rice Krispies instead of crackers and cut the chicken breasts into nuggets instead of strips.

CHICKEN FINGERS	**PLUM DIPPING SAUCE**
Each serving: (1/5 recipe)	Each serving: (1/5 recipe)

1	■	Starch choice	1/2	Sugars choice
3		Protein choices		

OVEN-BAKED CRISPY CHICKEN

1 whole	Cut-up chicken (or 8 pieces)	1 whole
125 ml	Corn flake crumbs	1/2 cup
10 ml	Garlic powder	2 tsp
10 ml	Seasoning salt	2 tsp
10 ml	Chili powder	2 tsp
2 ml	Pepper	1/2 tsp
25 ml	Parmesan cheese	2 tbsp
50 ml	2% Milk	1/4 cup

☺ ☺ ☺ ☺ Makes 4 servings

1. Preheat the oven to 180° (350°F). Spray a baking pan with vegetable oil spray.
2. Rinse the chicken pieces and remove all skin and visible fat. Pat them dry.
3. Cut the chicken breasts in half and cut the drumsticks and thighs apart at the joint (save the wings and back for another use). You should have 8 pieces of chicken.
4. In a plastic bag combine the corn flake crumbs, garlic powder, seasoning salt, chili powder, pepper, and parmesan cheese.
5. Dip the chicken pieces in the milk and then add them to the plastic bag, one at a time. Shake to coat with crumbs.
6. Place the chicken onto the baking pan and sprinkle with any remaining crumbs.
7. Bake for 45–50 minutes.

Did You Know?

Removing the skin from chicken cuts the fat by more than half!

Each serving: (2 pieces)

1		Starch choice
4		Protein choices

TEX'S TACOS

500 g	Ground turkey (or lean beef)	1 lb
125 ml	Chopped onion	1/2 cup
2 cloves	Garlic	2 cloves
50 ml	Ketchup	1/4 cup
25 ml	Chili powder	2 tbsp
5 ml	Salt	1 tsp
125 ml	Frozen corn	1/2 cup
250 ml	Garbanzo or kidney beans	1 cup
10	Taco shells	10
1	Large tomato, chopped	1
300 ml	Grated 'light' cheddar cheese	1 1/4 cups
500 ml	Shredded lettuce	2 cups
50 ml	Salsa	1/4 cup

☺ ☺ ☺ ☺ ☺ Makes 5 servings

1. Preheat the oven to 180° (350°F).
2. Fry the ground turkey in a large skillet until brown and crumbly (4–5 minutes). Add the chopped onion and garlic, cook until the onion is tender, about 2 minutes.
3. Drain and rinse the garbanzo or kidney beans and then mash them with a potato masher or fork.
4. Add the ketchup, chili powder, salt, corn, mashed beans and 50ml (1/4 cup) of water to the turkey mixture. Simmer for 10 minutes, stirring occasionally.
5. Meanwhile, place the taco shells on a baking sheet and bake at 180° (350°F) for 8–10 minutes.
6. While the filling and shells are cooking; shred the lettuce, chop the tomatoes and grate the cheese.
7. To serve: spoon the meat mixture into the taco shells and top with the grated cheese, shredded lettuce, tomato and salsa.

Each serving: (2 tacos)

2	■	Starch choices	3		Protein choices
1/2		Fruit & Vegetable choice	2	▲	Fats & Oils choices

GARDEN BURRITOS

1	Can (398ml/14 oz) black beans	1
1	Can (398ml/14 oz) kernel corn	1
1	Can (398ml/14 oz) Mexican style stewed tomatoes	1
15 ml	Fresh cilantro (optional)	1 tbsp
375 ml	Grated Monterey Jack cheese	1 1/2 cup
8 -22 cm	Flour tortillas	8 - 8"

☺ ☺ ☺ ☺ ☺ ☺ ☺ ☺ Makes 8 servings

1. Preheat the oven to 200° (400°F). Spray a shallow 3L (12"x18") quart baking dish with vegetable oil spray.
2. Drain and rinse the black beans; drain corn.
3. In a medium-sized mixing bowl combine the beans, corn, tomatoes, chopped cilantro, and cheese.
4. Divide evenly between the tortillas. Fold tortillas, making sure ends are tucked in burrito style.
5. Place the burritos in the prepared baking dish and bake at 200° (400°F) for 8 to 10 minutes

Did You Know?

Cilantro is a member of the parsley family that has an unusual taste. You will find it always listed as optional in this cookbook because not everybody likes it.

Each serving: (1 burrito)

1 1/2	Starch choices	1	Protein choice
1	Fruit & Vegetable choice	1	▲ Fats & Oils choice

CHILI CON CARNE

375 g	Extra-lean ground beef	3/4 lb
50 ml	Diced onion	1/4 cup
1	clove garlic, minced	1
50 ml	Chopped green pepper	1/4 cup
1	Can (398ml/14 oz) kidney beans, drained	1
1	Can (398ml/14 oz) diced or crushed tomatoes	1
15 ml	Chili powder	1 tbsp
15 ml	Cocoa	1 tbsp
15 ml	Splenda®	1 tbsp
15 ml	Vinegar	1 tbsp
5 ml	Pumpkin pie spice	1 tsp
2 ml	Salt	1/2 tsp

☺ ☺ ☺ ☺ Makes 4 servings

1. Cook ground beef in a medium-sized saucepan until brown (about 5 minutes). Stir often while it is cooking so that it is crumbly.
2. Add the diced onion, garlic, and green pepper and continue cooking for 2 minutes.
3. Stir in the kidney beans, tomatoes, chili powder, cocoa, Splenda®, vinegar, pumpkin pie spice and salt. Bring just to a boil.
4. Turn heat to low and simmer for 30 minutes or more. Add 50 ml (1/4 cup) of water if it becomes too thick.

Fun ways to eat chili…
With toast, in tacos, on pasta, on French fries, or on a baked potato with cheese and sour cream!

Each serving: (1/4 recipe)

| 1 | ■ Starch choice | 3 | Protein choices |
| 1/2 | Fruit & Vegetable choice | 1/2 | ▲ Fats & Oils choice |

REFRITO BURRITOS

125 ml	Chopped onion	1/2 cup
2	Cloves garlic, minced	2
50 ml	Diced green or red pepper	1/4 cup
1	Can (398ml/14 oz) refried beans	1
15 ml	Chopped Jalapeño pepper	1 tbsp
5 ml	Chili powder	1 tsp
1 ml	Cumin (optional)	1/4 tsp
6 – 22 cm	Tortillas	6–8"
375 ml	Grated part skim mozzarella cheese	1 1/2 cups
2	Green onions, chopped	2

☺ ☺ ☺ ☺ ☺ ☺ Makes 6 servings

1. Preheat the oven to 180° (350°F).
2. Place the chopped onion and garlic in a microwave-safe cooking dish, cover with plastic wrap and cook for one minute. Add the diced green pepper and continue cooking for 1 1/2 – 2 minutes, or until the onion is soft.
3. Meanwhile, in a medium-sized saucepan, heat the refried beans, Jalapeño pepper and spices. Add to the micro-cooked vegetables and heat for 2 minutes.
4. Spoon 1/6 of the bean mixture in the centre of each tortilla. Sprinkle with the cheese and green onions. Fold the lower edge up over the filling, fold in the ends and then roll up.
5. Place the burritos on an ungreased cookie sheet and bake at 180° (350°F) for 15–20 minutes.
6. Serve with salsa and 0.1% sour cream if desired.

Each serving: (1 burrito)

| 1 1/2 | ■ | Starch choices | 1/2 | ▲ | Fats & Oils choice |
| 1 1/2 | ⊘ | Protein choices | 1 | ++ | Extra choice |

HAWAIIAN CHILI

375 g	Ground turkey	3/4 lb
50 ml	Diced onion	1/4 cup
1	Clove garlic, minced	1
50 ml	Chopped green pepper	1/4 cup
1	Can (398ml/14 oz) stewed tomatoes	1
1	Can (156 ml/5.5 oz) tomato paste	1
1	Can (398ml/14 oz) kidney beans	1
45 ml	Soy sauce (low sodium)	3 tbsp
10 ml	Chili powder	2 tsp
10 ml	Splenda®	2 tsp
250 ml	Uncooked rice	1 cup
50 ml	Diced green onions (optional)	1/4 cup

☺ ☺ ☺ ☺ ☺ ☺ Makes 6 servings

1. Cook the ground turkey in a medium-sized saucepan, stirring often, until brown and crumbly.
2. Add the onion, garlic, and green pepper; cook for 2 minutes.
3. Stir in the remaining ingredients and bring just to a boil.
4. Reduce heat and simmer for 30 minutes. Add a little water if it becomes too thick.
5. Meanwhile, in a small saucepan, bring 500 ml (2 cups) of water to a boil. Add 2 ml (1/2 tsp) of salt and the rice. Cover tightly and simmer for 25 minutes.
6. To serve: divide chili on 125 ml (1/2 cup) rice per serving and sprinkle with green onions, if desired.

Each serving: (1/6 recipe)

2	■	Starch choices	2	⊘	Protein choices
1	◢	Fruit & Vegetable choice	1	++	Extra choice

SALMON & CHEDDAR MACARONI

250 ml	Elbow macaroni	1 cup
20 ml	Soft 'diet' margarine	4 tsp
50 ml	Finely chopped onion	1/4 cup
1	Clove garlic, minced (optional)	1
25 ml	Flour	2 tbsp
2 ml	Worcestershire sauce	1/2 tsp
375 ml	2% Milk	1 1/2 cups
150 ml	Grated 'light' cheddar cheese	2/3 cup
125 ml	'Light' sour cream	1/2 cup
2 ml	Salt & pepper	1/2 tsp
1	Can (213g/7.5 oz) salmon, drained	1
125 ml	Bread crumbs	1/2 cup

☺ ☺ ☺ ☺ Makes 4 servings

1. Cook the macaroni in 1 L (4 cups) of boiling salted water for 8 to 10 minutes. Drain carefully.
2. Melt 15ml (1 tbsp) margarine in a large saucepan. Sauté the onion and garlic in the margarine for 3 minutes. Stir in the flour. Add the Worcestershire and gradually stir in the milk with a whisk until smooth.
3. Cook over medium heat, stirring constantly, until the mixture comes to a boil and thickens. Remove from the heat.
4. Set aside 25ml (2 tbsp) of cheese; add the rest to the sauce and stir until melted. Stir in the sour cream, salt and pepper.
5. Flake the salmon with a fork and stir into the sauce. Stir in the cooked macaroni.
6. Preheat the oven to 180° (350°F). Spray a 2L (2 qt.) casserole lightly with vegetable oil spray and spoon in the macaroni mixture.
7. Combine the bread crumbs, 5 ml (1 tsp) melted margarine, and the reserved cheese. Sprinkle on top of the macaroni.
8. Bake uncovered at 180° (350°F) for 30 minutes.

Each serving: (1/4 recipe)

2	■	Starch choices	2		Protein choices
1	◆	2% Milk choice	1	▲	Fats & Oils choice

LASAGNA

12	Lasagna noodles	12
250 g	Ground turkey or lean beef	1/2 lb
5 ml	Vegetable or olive oil	1 tsp
1	Onion, chopped	1
2	Cloves garlic, minced	2
1/2	Chopped green pepper	1/2
1	Can (398 ml/14 oz) diced or crushed tomatoes	1
1	Can (156g/5.5 oz) tomato paste	1
250 g	Mushrooms, sliced	1/2 lb
5 ml each	Dried oregano and dried basil	1 tsp each
2 ml each	Salt and pepper	1/2 tsp each
500 ml	1% cottage cheese	2 cups
2	Egg whites	2
3	Green onions, minced	3
500 ml	Grated part-skim mozzarella	2 cups
25 ml	Parmesan cheese	2 tbsp

☺ ☺ ☺ ☺ ☺ ☺   ☺ ☺ Makes 6 or 8 servings

1. Brown the ground meat in a large heavy saucepan in 5 ml (1 tsp) of oil for 5 minutes (until no longer pink).
2. Add the chopped onion and garlic and continue cooking for 2 minutes. Add the green pepper and cook one minute more.
3. Stir in the tomatoes, tomato paste, mushrooms, and spices. Allow to simmer uncovered for 30 minutes more.
4. Meanwhile, boil the noodles according to package directions to 'al dente' (still firm but tender), do NOT overcook. Drain, rinse and set aside.
5. In a small mixing bowl, combine the cottage cheese, egg whites, and minced green onion.

continued on next page ...

LASAGNA
CONTINUED

To assemble lasagna:

1. Spread a little meat sauce in the bottom of a 3.5 L (9" x 13") lasagna pan. Top with four noodles overlapping them slightly.
2. Top with half of the cottage cheese mixture, then one-third of the tomato sauce. Sprinkle with 150 ml (2/3 cup) of mozzarella.
3. Repeat layers and top with remaining 4 noodles, remaining sauce and parmesan cheese.
4. Cover with foil and bake in 180° (350°F) oven for 40 minutes.
5. Remove foil, sprinkle with remaining 150ml (2/3 cup) mozzarella and bake, uncovered for 10 minutes.
6. Remove from oven and let sit 5 to 10 minutes before serving.

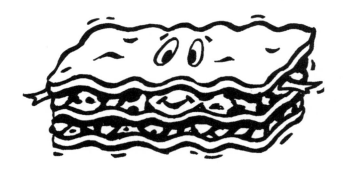

Each serving: (1/8 recipe)   Each serving: (1/6 recipe)

1	■	Starch choice	1 1/2	■	Starch choices
1	◆	Fruit & vegetable	1	◆	Fruit & vegetable
3 1/2	⊘	Protein choices	4 1/2	⊘	Protein choices

LASAGNA ROLL-UPS

12	Lasagna noodles	12
1	Package (284g/10 oz) frozen chopped broccoli	1
2	Green onions, minced	2
500 ml	1% cottage cheese	2 cups
50 ml	Parmesan cheese	1/4 cup
2 ml	Salt	1/2 tsp
1	Egg	1
500 ml	Prepared spaghetti sauce	2 cups
250 ml	Grated part-skim mozzarella	1 cup

☺ ☺ ☺ ☺ ☺ ☺ Makes 6 servings

1. Cook lasagna noodles according to package directions. Drain, rinse and set aside.
2. Meanwhile, put the broccoli in a microwave safe dish, cover with plastic wrap and cook for 3 minutes. Add the minced green onion and continue cooking for 1 to 2 minutes. Drain well and squeeze out the extra moisture with the back of a spoon.
3. Combine the cottage cheese, parmesan cheese, salt and egg in a medium-sized mixing bowl. Stir in the drained broccoli and green onions.
4. Preheat the oven to 180° (350°F).
5. Place the cooked noodles on wax paper. Evenly spread some cheese and broccoli mixture on each noodle. Roll up each noodle.
6. Using a 4 L (9" x 13") baking dish, spoon in about two-thirds of the spaghetti sauce. Arrange the rolled noodles with their seams down, on the sauce. Top with remaining sauce and cover with foil.
7. Bake for 25 minutes.
8. Uncover, sprinkle with mozzarella and continue baking until the cheese melts (10 minutes).

Each serving: (2 roll-ups)

2	■	Starch choices	2 1/2	⊘	Protein choices
1	◆	Fruit & vegetable choice	1/2	▲	Fats & Oils choice

SPAGHETTI & MEATBALL SKILLET

250 g	Lean ground beef	1/2 lb
25 ml	Bread crumbs	2 tbsp
1	Egg white	1
2 ml	Salt	1/2 tsp
250 ml	Sliced mushrooms	1 cup
125 ml	Chopped onion	1/2 cup
1	Clove garlic, minced	1
125 ml	Chopped green pepper	1/2 cup
1	Can (540ml/19 oz) diced tomatoes	1
250 ml	Water	1 cup
250 ml	Spaghetti in 4-5 cm (2" to 3") pieces	1 cup
5 ml	Italian seasoning	1 tsp
5 ml	salt	1 tsp
250 ml	Grated part skim mozzarella cheese	1 cup

☺ ☺ ☺ ☺ Makes 4 servings

1. In a medium-sized bowl, combine the egg, bread crumbs, salt and ground beef. Mix well (with your hands). Shape into 2.5 cm (1") meatballs.
2. In a large non-stick skillet, fry meatballs, turning often until browned (about 5 minutes). Remove the meatballs from the skillet with a slotted spoon and place them on paper towels.
3. Meanwhile, as the meatballs are cooking, chop the onions, garlic, and peppers. Slice the mushrooms.
4. In the skillet, sauté the mushrooms, garlic, onions, and peppers until the onions are tender. Return the meatballs to the skillet.
5. Add the tomatoes, water, Italian seasoning, spaghetti pieces and the salt. Bring to a boil.
6. Reduce heat, cover pan and simmer 20 minutes, stirring occasionally.
7. Add the cheese; stir until melted. Serve immediately.

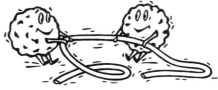

Each serving: (1/4 recipe)

1		Starch choice	3		Protein choices
1/2		Fruit & vegetable choice	1 1/2		Fats & Oils choices

SWEET & SOUR MEATBALLS

500 g	Extra lean ground beef	1 lb
25 ml	Bread crumbs	2 tbsp
1	Egg white	1
2 ml each	Salt & pepper	1/2 tsp each
1	Onion, chopped	1
2	Carrots, sliced	2
250 ml	Pineapple chunks, in juice	1 cup
125 ml	Water	1/2 cup
45 ml	Splenda®	3 tbsp
45 ml	Cider vinegar	3 tbsp
25 ml	Cornstarch	2 tbsp
25 ml	Soy sauce (low sodium)	2 tbsp
15 ml	Ketchup	1 tbsp
125 ml	Chopped green pepper (chunks)	1/2 cup
500 ml	Hot cooked rice	2 cups

☺ ☺ ☺ ☺ Makes 4 servings

1. In a medium-sized bowl, combine the bread crumbs, egg white, salt and pepper. Add the ground beef and mix well. Shape into 24 meatballs.
2. In a large non-stick skillet, heat 5 ml (1 tbsp) vegetable oil. Fry the meatballs until brown on all sides (about 5 minutes).
3. With a slotted spoon, remove the meatballs and place on paper towels.
4. In the same skillet, stir-fry the onion and carrots, at medium heat for 3 minutes.
5. Drain the pineapple, reserving the juice. Set the pineapple aside. Combine the reserved juice, water, Splenda®, vinegar, cornstarch, ketchup, and soy sauce in a small bowl. Stir until the cornstarch is dissolved.
6. Pour the juice mixture into the skillet with the onions and carrots, and cook, stirring until the sauce is clear and thickened.
7. Return the meatballs to the pan. Cover and simmer gently for 15 minutes. Uncover, add the pineapple and green pepper chunks; cook for 5 minutes.
8. Serve with hot rice.

Each serving: (1/4 recipe)

3		Starch choices	3 1/2		Protein choices
1 1/2		Fruit & vegetable choices	2	▲	Fats & Oils choices

FETTUCCINI ALFREDO

1	Package (350g) fresh fettuccini	1
20 ml	Butter	4 tsp
125 ml	1% cottage cheese	1/2 cup
125 ml	2% milk	1/2 cup
75 ml	Parmesan cheese	1/3 cup
	Salt & pepper to taste	
	Fresh chopped parsley (optional)	

☺ ☺ ☺ ☺ ☺ ☺ Makes 6 servings

1. In a large pot of boiling salted water, cook the pasta for 3 minutes, (until tender but firm). It is best with fresh pasta but if you are using dried pasta, cook according to package directions.
2. Meanwhile, mix the cottage cheese, milk, parmesan cheese, salt and pepper in a blender or food processor until smooth.
3. Drain the pasta, then return the pasta to the pot. Over low heat, toss the pasta with the butter until melted. Add the milk and cheese mixture, stir until the pasta is coated and hot.
4. Serve immediately, sprinkled with fresh parsley and more parmesan cheese (15 ml [1 tbsp] = 1 protein + 1 fats & oils choice).

Each serving: (1/6 recipe)

2	■	Starch choices
1	⊘	Protein choice
1/2	▲	Fats & Oils choice

DESSERTS

Page		Carbohydrates	Proteins	Fats	Calories	Kilojoules
102	**Strawberry Delights**	10	2	2	63	265
103	**Fruit On A Cloud**	33	4	5	222	932
104	**Peach Or Cherry Cobbler**	31	3	4	163	685
105	**Peanut Butter Apple Crisp**	41	4	4	205	861
106	**Brownie Sundae Supreme**	37	9	10	268	1126
107	**Chocolate Sauce**	5	2	0	36	151
108	**Raspberry Brownie Parfait**	38	7	13	287	1205
108	**Fresh Fruit Parfait**	40	5	2	185	777
109	**Frozen Lemon Pie**	51	5	10	300	1260
110	**Chocolate Bavarian Pie**	24	5	6	165	693
111	**Sour Cream & Berry Pie**	29	5	8	207	869
112	**Strawberry Mousse Pie**	25	4	7	169	710
113	**Angel Tunnel Cake**	40	3	3	196	823
114	**Fruit Filled Angel Tunnel Cake**	42	5	3	215	903
115	**Spiced Angel Food Cake**	31	3	0	132	554
116	**Strawberry Rainbow Cake**	24	2	4	132	554
117	**Ice Cream Fantasy Cake**	38	6	9	254	1067
118	**Quick Chocolate Mousse**	9	2	4	74	311
119	**Frozen Flying Saucers**	15	2	3	102	428
120	**Phyllo Fruit Pie**	39	1	2	163	685
121	**Peppermint Angel Cake**	45	5	1	201	844
122	**Spicy Apple Cupcakes**	21	2	5	130	546

Nutritional Analysis (per Serving)

STRAWBERRY DELIGHTS

24	Large strawberries	24
1	Pkg (125g/3oz) 'light' cream cheese	1
25 ml	Splenda®	2 tbsp
7 ml	Lemon juice	1 1/2 tsp
50 ml	Chocolate sprinkles	1/4 cup

☺ ☺ ☺ ☺ ☺ ☺ ☺ ☺ Makes 8 servings

1. Let the cream cheese warm to room temperature. Wash the strawberries and pat dry with a paper towel.
2. In a small bowl, combine the softened cream cheese, the Splenda®, and the lemon juice. Blend well.
3. Holding each strawberry by its leaf, dip the bottom half of the strawberry into the cream cheese mixture, coating it well. Then dip it in the chocolate sprinkles and set on wax paper.
4. Repeat until all the strawberries are done.
   Arrange the berries on a serving plate and refrigerate until serving time.

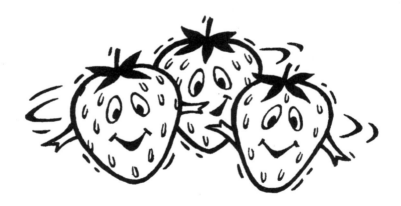

Each serving: (3 berries)

1	◆	Fruit & vegetable choice
1/2	▲	Fats & Oils choice

FRUIT ON A CLOUD

1	Pkg (125g/3oz) 'light' cream cheese	1
250 ml	Cool Whip® 'Light'	1 cup
250 ml	Miniature marshmallows	1 cup
500 ml	Fresh fruit such as: raspberries, blueberries, grapes, and nectarines (sliced)	2 cups

☺ ☺ ☺ ☺ Makes 4 servings

1. Line a cookie sheet with waxed paper.
2. In a medium-sized mixing bowl, beat the cream cheese with an electric mixer until it is light and fluffy.
3. Add the Cool Whip® 'Light' and beat until smooth, about 2 minutes. Stir in the marshmallows.
4. To make clouds, spoon the cream cheese mixture in 4 mounds onto the waxed paper. Spread each mound into an 8 cm (3 inch) circle with the back of a spoon and make a deep well in the centre of each circle, building up the sides.
5. Freeze for 2-3 hours.
6. Remove the clouds from the freezer and place each on individual serving plates. Let them stand at room temperature for 15 minutes.
7. Meanwhile, combine the fruit in a small bowl.
8. Spoon 125 ml (1/2 cup) of the fruit into the centre of each cloud and serve immediately.

Just For FUN...

This recipe can be varied by using your favourite fruit. It can also be varied by drizzling 'calorie reduced' sundae topping over the fruit. Try fresh sliced strawberries and chocolate sauce!

Each serving: (1 'cloud')

1 1/2	Fruit & vegetable choices		1/2	Protein choice	
1 1/2	✳ Sugars choices		1/2	Fats & Oil choice	

PEACH OR CHERRY COBBLER

750 ml	Cherries, berries or sliced fresh peaches	3 cups
50 ml	Granulated sugar	1/4 cup
15 ml	Cornstarch	1 tbsp
50 ml	Splenda®	1/4 cup
50 ml	Water	1/4 cup

TOPPING:

1	Egg	1
15 ml	Margarine	1 tbsp
15 ml	Milk	1 tbsp
125 ml	Flour	1/2 cup
50 ml	Splenda®	1/4 cup
2 ml	Baking powder	1/2 tsp
1 ml	Salt	1/4 tsp

☺ ☺ ☺ ☺ ☺ ☺ Makes 6 servings

1. Preheat the oven to 190° (375°F).
2. Combine the granulated sugar and the cornstarch; toss with the fruit and 50 ml (1/4 cup) of Splenda® in a medium-sized saucepan. Add the water and stir to mix. Bring to a boil over medium heat, stirring frequently. Simmer for 5 minutes.
3. Meanwhile, beat the egg and the margarine together with an electric mixer, add the milk.
4. In a separate bowl, stir together the flour, 50 ml (1/4 cup) Splenda®, the baking powder, and salt. Beat the flour mixture into the egg mixture.
5. Spread the hot fruit into a baking dish, and drop the batter by spoonfuls evenly over top of the fruit. Sprinkle with a mixture of 2 ml (1/2 tsp) cinnamon and 15 ml (1 tbsp) sugar.
6. Bake 25-30 minutes. (Yummy served with frozen yogurt or ice milk.)

Each serving: (1/6 recipe)

1/2	■	Starch choice	1	✳	Sugar choice
1	◢	Fruit & vegetable choice	1	▲	Fats & Oils choice

PEANUT BUTTER APPLE CRISP

FRUIT LAYER:

1 L	Peeled and sliced apples	4 cups
75 ml	Peanut butter chips	1/3 cup
125 ml	Splenda®	1/2 cup
25 ml	Flour	2 tbsp

TOPPING:

150 ml	Quick rolled oats	2/3 cup
125 ml	Flour	1/2 cup
50 ml	Splenda®	1/4 cup
25 ml	Brown sugar	2 tbsp
2 ml	Cinnamon	1/2 tsp
50 ml	Soft 'diet' margarine	1/4 cup

☺ ☺ ☺ ☺ ☺ ☺ ☺ ☺ Makes 8 servings

1. Preheat the oven to 180° (350°F). Spray a 23 cm (9 inch) square baking pan with vegetable oil spray.
2. In a large bowl, stir together the apples, peanut butter chips, 125 ml (1/2 cup) Splenda®, and 25 ml (2 tbsp) of flour. Spread into the prepared pan.
3. In a medium bowl, combine the topping ingredients until crumbly. Sprinkle over the apple layer.
4. Bake for 40-45 minutes at 180° (350°F) or until the apples are tender.
5. Serve warm, topped with 15 ml (1 tbsp) of Cool Whip® 'Light' or ice milk, if desired.

Did you know?

Read the labels on the peanut butter chips. Some have twice as many grams of fat as others.

Each serving: (1/8 recipe)

1/2		Starch choice	1		Sugars choice
2		Fruit & vegetable choices	1		Fats & Oils choice

BROWNIE SUNDAE SUPREME

8	Chocolate brownies (see page 41)	8
500 ml	Vanilla ice milk (1%)	2 cups
50 ml	Chocolate sauce (see page 107)	1/4 cup

Optional toppings:

50 ml	Cool Whip® 'Light'	1/4 cup
4	Maraschino cherries OR	4
20 ml	Chopped nuts	4 tsp

☺ ☺ ☺ ☺ Makes 4 servings

For each sundae:

1. Place two chocolate brownies in each dessert dish.
2. Scoop 125 ml (1/2 cup) of ice milk on top of the brownies.
3. Drizzle ice milk with 15 ml (1 tbsp) of chocolate sauce.
4. If desired, top with 15 ml (1 tbsp) of Cool Whip® 'Light' or a maraschino cherry or 5 ml (1 tsp) chopped nuts and serve.

Did you know?

25 ml (2 tbsp) Cool Whip® 'Light' = 1 Extra choice
1 Maraschino cherry = 1 Extra choice and
5 ml (1 tsp) of chopped nuts = 1 Extra choice
But they are not free foods and should be limited to 2 per day.

Each serving: (1/4 recipe)

1	■ Starch choice	1/2	⬭ Protein choice
1	◆ 1% Milk choice	1 1/2	▲ Fats & Oils choices
1 1/2	✱ Sugars choices		

CHOCOLATE SAUCE

15 ml	Cornstarch	1 tbsp
50 ml	Unsweetened cocoa powder	1/4 cup
50 ml	Water	1/4 cup
175 ml	Evaporated skim milk	3/4 cup
125 ml	Splenda®	1/2 cup
5 ml	Vanilla	1 tsp

☺ ☺ ☺ ☺ ☺ ☺ ☺ ☺ Makes 8 servings

1. Combine the cocoa and the cornstarch in a small saucepan.
2. Whisk in 50 ml (1/4 cup) of water until it is smooth.
3. Whisk in milk and cook over low heat, stirring often until the mixture comes to a boil.
4. Cook one minute more, until thickened (it will thicken more as it cools).
5. Remove from heat, stir in the Splenda® and vanilla.
6. Allow to cool. Store in refrigerator for up to 3 days.

Each serving: (25 ml [2 tbsp])

 1/2 Skim milk choice

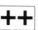 1 ++ Extra choice

PARFAIT

RASPBERRY BROWNIE PARFAIT

6	Chocolate brownies (see page 41)	6
500 ml	Frozen raspberry yogurt	2 cups
125 ml	Fresh raspberries	1/2 cup
50 ml	Cool Whip® 'Light'	1/4 cup

☺ ☺ ☺ ☺ Makes 4 servings

1.   Cut the brownies into little pieces (you will use 1 1/2 brownies for each parfait).
2   In dessert dishes (or parfait glasses), layer 50 ml (1/4 cup) of the frozen yogurt, 1/2 of the brownie squares, and 15 ml (1 tbsp) of fresh raspberries; repeat layers.
3.   Top each parfait with 15 ml (1 tbsp) of Cool Whip® 'Light' and a "pretty" raspberry.

FRESH FRUIT PARFAIT

500 ml	Vanilla ice milk (1%)	2 cups
500 ml	Fresh fruit (pineapple, kiwi, strawberries, blueberries, oranges)	2 cups
50 ml	Cool Whip® 'Light'	1/4 cup

☺ ☺ ☺ ☺ Makes 4 servings

1.   Prepare the fresh fruit by chopping it into small chunks.
2   In dessert dishes (or parfait glasses) layer 50 ml (1/4 cup) of ice milk and 50 ml (1/4 cup) of diced fruit; repeat layers.
3.   Top with 15 ml (1 tbsp) of Cool Whip® 'Light'.

RASPBERRY		**FRESH FRUIT**	
Each serving: (1/4 recipe)		Each serving: (1/4 recipe)	
1/2	■ Starch choice	1 1/2	◆ Fruit & Vegetable
1	◆ 1 % Milk choice	1	◆ 1% Milk choice
2	✳ Sugars choices	1 1/2	✳ Sugars choices
1/2	⊘ Protein choice		
2	▲ Fats & Oils choices		

FROZEN LEMON PIE

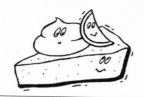

1	Can (175 ml/6 oz) frozen lemonade	1
750 ml	Vanilla frozen yogurt	3 cups
500 ml	Frozen Cool Whip® 'Light'	2 cups
1	Graham wafer crust	1
	Fresh lemon slices for garnish	

☺ ☺ ☺ ☺ ☺ ☺ ☺ ☺ Makes 8 servings

1. Thaw the lemonade concentrate slightly.
2. Put the semi-frozen concentrate into a large mixing bowl and beat for 30 seconds. Gradually stir in the frozen yogurt.
3. Fold in 375 ml (1 1/2 cups) of the Cool Whip® 'Light' and stir until blended and smooth.
4. Freeze until mixture will mound (about 30 minutes).
5. Spoon into the prepared pie crust and freeze until firm, at least 4 hours.
6. Garnish each serving with 15 ml (1 tbsp) Cool Whip® 'Light' and lemon slices.

GRAHAM WAFER CRUST:

175 ml	Graham wafer crumbs	3/4 cup
45 ml	Melted margarine	3 tbsp
1 ml	Cinnamon	1/4 tsp
1 ml	Nutmeg	1/4 tsp

1. Combine the graham wafer crumbs, margarine, cinnamon, and nutmeg in a small mixing bowl.
2. Press into a 1L (9 inch) pie plate.
3. Refrigerate for 2 hours before filling.

Each serving: (1/8 pie)

1	■	Starch choice	3		Sugars choices
1/2	◆	Skim milk choice	2	▲	Fats & Oils choices

CHOCOLATE BAVARIAN PIE

1	Chocolate 'Oreo®' pie shell	1
1	Envelope unflavoured gelatin	1
375 ml	2% Milk	1 1/2 cups
150 ml	Splenda®	2/3 cups
50 ml	Unsweetened cocoa powder	1/4 cup
2 ml	Vanilla extract	1/2 tsp
125 ml	'No-fat' plain yogurt	1/2 cup

STRAWBERRY COOL WHIP:

125 ml	Strawberries	1/2 cup
250 ml	Cool Whip® 'Light'	1 cup

☺ ☺ ☺ ☺ ☺ ☺ ☺ ☺ Makes 8 servings

1. Pour 250 ml (1 cup) of milk into a medium-sized saucepan and sprinkle with the gelatin; let stand for 2 minutes.
2. Combine the Splenda® and cocoa, whisk into the milk and gelatin mixture.
3. Cook over medium heat, whisking constantly, until the mixture boils. Cook and stir for 1 minute.
4. Remove from the heat and stir in the remaining 125 ml (1/2 cup) milk and the vanilla. Let cool to room temperature.
5. Stir in the yogurt and then refrigerate until the mixture begins to set.
6. Spoon into the Oreo® pie shell; chill until set (4 hours or more).
7. To prepare the Strawberry Cool Whip; if frozen, thaw and drain berries well, wash and pat them dry if fresh.
8. Puree the berries in a food processor. Fold into the Cool Whip® 'Light'. Serve on the chilled and set pie.

Each serving: (1/8 pie)

1/2		Starch choice	1 1/2	✳	Sugars choices
1/2	◆	2% Milk choice	1	▲	Fats & Oils choice

SOUR CREAM & BERRY PIE

1	Graham wafer crust (see pg.109)	1
45 ml	Cornstarch	3 tbsp
1	Package unflavoured gelatin	1
125 ml	Splenda®	1/2 cup
375 ml	2% Milk	1 1/2 cup
250 ml	0.1% sour cream	1 cup
125 ml	'No-fat' plain yogurt	1/2 cup
5 ml	Vanilla extract	1 tsp
750 ml	Raspberries, blueberries and sliced small strawberries	3 cups

☺ ☺ ☺ ☺ ☺ ☺ ☺ ☺ Makes 8 servings

1. In a medium-sized saucepan, combine the cornstarch and gelatin; stir in the Splenda®. Add the milk.
2. Cook and stir over medium heat until thickened and bubbly. Continue cooking and stirring for 2 minutes. Cool slightly.
3. While the mixture is cooling, combine the sour cream and yogurt, in a medium-sized bowl.
4. Slowly stir the warm milk mixture into the sour cream mixture and add the vanilla extract. Cover and chill for 1 hour, stirring once or twice.
5. Wash the berries and pat them dry with a paper towel. Reserve 125 ml (1/2 cup) of berries for garnish and fold the rest into the sour cream mixture.
6. Spoon the sour cream and berry mixture into the crust and garnish with the reserved berries.
7. Cover and chill for 4 to 6 hours.

Each serving: (1/8 pie)

1	■ Starch choice	1/2	2% Milk choice	
1	Fruit & Vegetable choice	1 1/2	Fats & Oils choices	

STRAWBERRY MOUSSE PIE

150 ml	Boiling water	2/3 cup
1	Package 'no sugar added' strawberry gelatin	1
125 ml	Cold water	1/2 cup
	Ice cubes	
500 ml	Cool Whip® 'Light'	2 cups
125 ml	'No-fat' plain yogurt	1/2 cup
1	Graham wafer crust (see pg.109)	1
250 ml	Sliced strawberries	1 cup

☺ ☺ ☺ ☺ ☺ ☺ ☺ ☺   Makes 8 servings

1. Pour the jello powder into a medium-sized mixing bowl. Stir in the boiling water. Stir for 2 minutes until all the jello is dissolved.
2. Mix together the cold water and enough ice to make 250 ml (1 cup). Stir into the jello until it is slightly thickened and the ice is melted.
3. Stir in 375 ml (11/2 cups) Cool Whip® 'Light' and the yogurt, mix until smooth.
4. Fold in 125 ml (1/2 cup) sliced strawberries.
5. Refrigerate for 10 minutes or until mixture begins to set. Spoon into the graham wafer pie crust.
6. Refrigerate for 4 hours or until firm. Garnish with the remaining 125 ml (1/2 cup) sliced fresh strawberries and 125 ml (1/2 cup) Cool Whip 'Light'.

Just For FUN...

Use your favourite fruit flavoured gelatin and fruit, for example, try orange with mandarin oranges, or raspberry with fresh raspberries...

Each serving: (1/8 pie)

1	■	Starch choice	1/2	✳	Sugars choice
1/2	◢	Fruit & Vegetable	1 1/2	▲	Fats & Oils choices

ANGEL TUNNEL CAKE

1	Package Angel Food cake mix	1
750 ml	Cool Whip® 'Light'	3 cups
375 ml	2% milk	1 1/2 cups
1	Package (10g) 'no sugar added' chocolate pudding mix	1
25 ml	Unsweetened cocoa powder	2 tbsp

☺ ☺ ☺ ☺ ☺ ☺ ☺ ☺ ☺ ☺ ☺ ☺ Makes 12 servings

1. Bake the Angel Food cake following the instructions on the package. Let it cool on a wire rack, inverted and in the pan.
2. When the cake is completely cool, remove it from the pan and slice a 2.5 cm (1 inch) layer off the top of the cake. Gently hollow out a trench in the cake 4 cm (11/2 inch) wide and 5 cm (2 inches) deep.
3. Cut the cake from out of the trench into small pieces.
4. Beat the milk and the pudding mix together in a large mixing bowl for 2 minutes.
5. Stir 250 ml (1 cup) of the Cool Whip® 'Light' and the reserved cake pieces into the pudding. Fill the trench with the pudding mixture and replace the top of the cake.
6. Sift the cocoa into the remaining Cool Whip® 'Light' and stir gently until it is smooth.
7. Frost the cake with the chocolate Cool Whip® 'Light' and chill until it is set (at least 4 hours or overnight).

Variation next page...

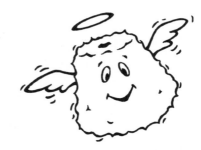

Each serving: (1/12 cake)

1		Starch choice
2 1/2	✳	Sugars choices
1/2	▲	Fats & Oils choice

FRUIT FILLED ANGEL TUNNEL CAKE

1	Package Angel Food cake mix	1
1	Package 'calorie reduced' lemon mousse mix	1
375 ml	2% milk	1 1/2cups
500 ml	Cool Whip® 'Light'	2 cups
250 ml	Fresh fruit (eg., strawberries, blueberries, kiwi)	1 cup

☺ ☺ ☺ ☺ ☺ ☺ ☺ ☺ ☺ ☺ ☺ ☺ Makes 12 servings

1. Bake the cake and hollow out as for Angel Tunnel Cake.
2. Beat the lemon mousse mix and the 2% milk in a medium-sized mixing bowl for 2 minutes.
3. Fold in 125 ml (1/2 cup) of Cool Whip® 'Light', the cut up fresh fruit and the cake pieces.
4. Fill the trench in the Angel Food cake with the fruit mixture instead of the chocolate pudding mixture.
5. Frost with 375 ml (11/2 cups) Cool Whip® 'Light' and chill for 4 hours or more.

It is hard to cut an Angel Food cake because it is sticky. Try using a wet knife with a serrated edge, and use your fingers to help hollow out the trench.

Each serving: (1/12 cake)

1	Starch choice		2	Sugars choices	
1/2	Fruit & Vegetable choice		1/2	Fats & Oils choice	

SPICED ANGEL FOOD CAKE

1	Package white Angel Food cake mix	1
5 ml	Cinnamon	1 tsp
5 ml	Ground ginger	1 tsp
2 ml	Nutmeg	1/2 tsp

Cran-apple topping:

4	Red apples (eg., Macintosh)	4
125 ml	Orange juice	1/2 cup
25 ml	Brown sugar	2 tbsp
10 ml	Cornstarch	2 tsp
75 ml	Splenda®	1/3 cup
5 ml	Cinnamon	1 tsp
50 ml	Water	1/4 cup
250 ml	Cranberries	1 cup

☺ ☺ ☺ ☺ ☺ ☺ ☺ ☺ ☺ ☺ ☺ ☺ ☺ ☺ ☺ ☺ Makes 16 servings

1. Add the cinnamon, ginger and nutmeg to the dry cake mix and then prepare and bake the cake following the directions on the package. Let it cool in the pan, inverted on a wire rack.
2. For cran-apple topping:
   Remove the cores and thinly slice the apples. Put them in a large skillet.
3. In a small mixing bowl, stir together the orange juice, brown sugar and cornstarch until smooth. Add the Splenda®, cinnamon and water.
4. Pour the orange juice mixture over the apples and cook over medium heat until the juice starts to bubble, stirring occasionally.
5. Reduce the heat to simmer and add the cranberries; simmer 10-15 minutes more or until the berries pop.
6. Serve the warm sauce over slices of the cake.

Each serving: (1/16 cake)

1	■	Starch choice
1/2		Fruit & Vegetable choice
1		Sugars choice

STRAWBERRY RAINBOW CAKE

1	Package white cake mix	1
1	Package 'no sugar added' strawberry gelatin	1
250 ml	Boiling water	1 cup
125 ml	Cold water	1/2 cup
500 ml	Cool Whip® 'Light'	2 cups
20	Strawberries	20

☺☺☺☺☺☺☺☺☺☺ Makes 20 servings
☺☺☺☺☺☺☺☺☺☺

1. Bake the cake mix in a 4L (9 x 13") pan according to the package instructions. Let it cool for 10 minutes.
2. Remove the cake from the pan and let it cool completely on a wire rack. Wash the pan.
3. In a medium-sized mixing bowl, dissolve the jello powder in the boiling water. Add the cold water and let it cool to room temperature.
4. When the cake is cool, put it back into the clean pan and prick the cake with a big serving fork at 1 cm (1/2 inch) intervals.
5. Pour the cooled jello carefully over the cake. Refrigerate for 3 to 4 hours.
6. Dip the pan into warm water and then invert onto a serving plate and remove the pan.
7. Frost the top and sides of the cake with Cool Whip® 'Light'.
8. Mark the frosting into 20 even pieces and garnish each square with a sliced strawberry.

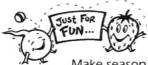

Make seasonal Rainbow cakes ... heart-shaped and pink for valentine's day, tree-shaped and green for Christmas. Add food colouring to the Cool Whip to match your design

Each serving: (1/20 cake)

1/2		Starch choice
1 1/2		Sugars choices
1/2		Fats & Oils choice

ICE CREAM FANTASY CAKE

15	Chocolate wafers	15
25 ml	Melted margarine	2 tbsp
1 L	Vanilla ice milk (1%)	4 cups
1	Recipe 'quick' chocolate mousse	1
1 L	Frozen raspberry yogurt	4 cups
250 ml	Cool Whip® 'Light'	1 cup
14	Strawberries or maraschino cherries	14
50 ml	'Calorie reduced' chocolate sundae sauce	1/2 cup

Optional: Chopped peanuts (25 ml [2 tbsp])

☺ ☺ ☺ ☺ ☺ ☺ ☺ ☺ ☺ ☺ ☺ ☺ ☺ ☺ Makes 14 servings

1. Grind the chocolate wafers into crumbs in a food processor or by crushing the wafers between two sheets of wax paper with a rolling pin.
2. Mix the chocolate crumbs with the melted margarine and press into the bottom of a 23 cm (9 inch) springform pan. Refrigerate to cool.
3. Allow the vanilla ice milk to soften slightly at room temperature. Spoon the soft ice milk onto the chocolate crumb crust and spread evenly. Freeze until solid.
4. Spread the chocolate mousse (SEE NEXT PAGE) over the frozen vanilla ice milk. Freeze again.
5. Scoop the frozen raspberry yogurt into nice round balls and arrange over the frozen chocolate mousse layer, covering it completely.
6. Pipe or spoon the Cool Whip® 'Light' decoratively around the outside edge of the cake top. Freeze if making ahead.
7. To serve: drizzle the cake top with chocolate syrup, sprinkle with chopped nuts and garnish with whole strawberries.
8. Remove the sides of springform pan, cut into 14 wedges and serve.

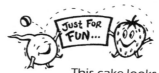

JUST FOR FUN...

This cake looks spectacular with sparklers for a special party!

Each serving: (1/14 cake)

1/2	Starch choice	2 1/2	Sugars choices
1	1% Milk choice	1 1/2	Fats & Oils choices

QUICK
CHOCOLATE MOUSSE

1	Package (10g) 'no sugar added' instant chocolate pudding	1
375 ml	2% milk	1 1/2 cups
500 ml	Cool Whip® 'Light'	2 cups

☺ ☺ ☺ ☺ ☺ ☺ ☺ ☺ ☺   Makes 8 servings

1.   Beat the chocolate pudding mix into the cold milk for 1 minute.
2.   Fold in the Cool Whip® 'Light'.

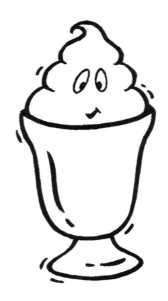

Each serving: (1/8 recipe)

1/2		2 % Milk choice
1/2		Sugars choice
1		Fats & Oils choice

FROZEN FLYING SAUCERS

1	Envelope 'low calorie' dessert topping mix	1
50 ml	2% milk	1/4 cup
1	Package (10 g) 'no sugar added' instant chocolate pudding mix	1
375 ml	2% milk	1 1/2 cups
36	Plain chocolate wafers	36

☺ ☺ ☺ ☺ ☺ ☺ ☺ ☺ ☺   Makes 18 servings
☺ ☺ ☺ ☺ ☺ ☺ ☺ ☺ ☺

1. Prepare the dessert topping with 50 ml (1/4 cup) of milk, following the directions on the package.
2. Stir the 375 ml (1 1/2 cups) milk and the pudding mix into the dessert topping. Beat on high speed with an electric mixer for 2 minutes, scraping the sides of the bowl occasionally with a rubber spatula.
3. Line a cookie sheet with wax paper and arrange 18 chocolate wafers in a single layer on the cookie sheet.
4. Spoon the chocolate pudding mixture onto the 18 chocolate wafers. Top with the remaining wafers, pressing lightly and smoothing around the edges with a knife, if necessary.
5. Freeze until firm, at least 3 hours. Store in a covered container in the freezer.

Each serving: (1 sandwich)

1/2	■	Starch choice
1	✱	Sugars choice
1/2	▲	Fats & Oils choice

PHYLLO FRUIT PIE

8	Apples (Granny Smith or cooking), pears or peaches	8
75 ml	Apple juice	1/3 cup
75 ml	Brown sugar	1/3 cup
75 ml	Splenda®	1/3 cup
45 ml	Flour	3 tbsp
25 ml	Lemon juice	2 tbsp
5 ml	Cinnamon	1 tsp
2 ml	Ginger	1/2 tsp
1 ml	Nutmeg	1/4 tsp
4	Sheets phyllo pastry	4
15 ml	Butter	1 tbsp
15 ml	Sugar	1 tbsp

☺ ☺ ☺ ☺ ☺ ☺ ☺ ☺   Makes 8 servings

1. Peel, core, and quarter the apples.
2. Cut each quarter into 1cm (1/2 inch) slices. Put apple slices into a heavy saucepan.
3. Stir the apple juice, brown sugar, Splenda®, flour, lemon juice, and spices together. Add to the apples and stir to coat.
4. Cover and cook for 20 minutes, (or until tender) stirring occasionally.
5. Preheat oven to 200° (400°F).
6. Spoon hot apple mixture into a 25cm (10 inch) pie plate. Let cool slightly.
7. Spread out one sheet of phyllo. Dot with 1/4 of the butter and sprinkle with 1/4 of the sugar. Fold the long end to make it square.
8. Lay another sheet of phyllo crosswise over the first, dot with butter and sugar, and fold to make it square. Continue with all the phyllo sheets.
9. Place the phyllo stack onto the pie filling. Dot with remaining butter and sprinkle with sugar.
10. Gather the edge of the phyllo to form a ruffle. Spray the ruffle with vegetable oil spray. Cut slits into the phyllo top to allow steam to escape.
11. Bake for 15 minutes, or until phyllo is golden.

Tip: Phyllo is a delicate Greek pastry that you can find ready-to-use in the frozen food section of the supermarket.

Each serving: (1/8 pie)

1/2		Starch choice	1	✳	Sugars choice
2	◢	Fruit & vegetable choices	1/2	▲	Fats & Oils choice

PEPPERMINT ANGEL CAKE

1 pkg	White Angel Food cake mix	1 pkg
50 ml	Peppermint candies	1/4 cup
125 ml	'Calorie reduced' chocolate sundae topping or chocolate sauce (see page 107)	1/2 cup

☺ ☺ ☺ ☺ ☺ ☺ ☺ ☺ ☺ ☺ ☺ ☺   Makes 12 servings

1. Crush the candies in a food processor or by smashing between tea towels.
2. Prepare cake mix according to package instructions. Stir one half of the candies into the cake mix. Pour into tube pan and cut through cake batter with a knife.
3. Bake according to package instructions. Invert immediately to cool. When completely cool remove from pan.
4. To serve drizzle the chocolate sauce on the top of the cake and sprinkle with the remaining candies

Each serving: (1/12 cake)

1		Starch choice
3		Sugars choices

SPICY APPLE CUPCAKES

50 ml	Margarine	1/4 cup
50 ml	White sugar	1/4 cup
50 ml	Brown sugar	1/4 cup
1	egg	1
2 ml	Vanilla	1/2 tsp
250 ml	Flour	1 cup
50 ml	Splenda®	1/4 cup
2 ml	Baking powder	1/2 tsp
2 ml	Baking soda	1/2 tsp
5 ml	Pumpkin pie spice	1 tsp
2 ml	Salt	1/2 tsp
125 ml	Unsweetened applesauce	1/2 cup

☺ ☺ ☺ ☺ ☺ ☺ ☺ ☺☺ ☺   Makes 10 servings

1. Preheat oven to 350°. Put 10 paper baking cups in a muffin pan (or spray with vegetable oil spray).
2. Cream the margarine and sugars together with a wooden spoon or in an electric mixer. Beat in the eggs and vanilla.
3. In a separate bowl mix together the flour, Splenda®, baking powder, baking soda, pumpkin pie spice and salt. Combine with the margarine mixture. Mix in the applesauce.
4. Fill the muffin tins half full.
5. Bake at 350° for 20-25 minutes.

Each serving: (1 muffin)

1	■	Starch choice
1/2	✳	Sugars choice
1	▲	Fats & Oils choice

INDEX

NOTES

KID'S CHOICE
COOKBOOK

ORDER FORM

Order **KID'S CHOICE COOKBOOK** at $14.95 per book
plus $4.00 (total order) for shipping and handling.

Number of books	_____ @ $14.95	=	_____
Postage and handling		=	$ 4.00
Subtotal	_____	=	_____
In Canada add 7% GST	_____	=	_____
Total enclosed	_____	=	_____

U.S. and international orders payable in U.S. funds.
Prices are subject to change.

Name: _____

Street: _____

City: _____ Prov./State _____

Country: _____ Zip code _____

Make Cheque or money order payable to: **PicNics Publishing**
P.O. Box 2461, Sechelt
British Columbia, Canada
V0N 3A0

For large volume purchases, contact: **PicNics Publishing.**
Fax: (604) 885-4375
Or fax: 1-800-947-5577
Please allow for 2 - 3 weeks delivery.

KID'S CHOICE
COOKBOOK

ORDER FORM

Order **KID'S CHOICE COOKBOOK** at $14.95 per book
plus $4.00 (total order) for shipping and handling.

Number of books	_____ @ $14.95	=	_____
Postage and handling		=	$ 4.00
Subtotal	_____	=	_____
In Canada add 7% GST	_____	=	_____
Total enclosed	_____	=	_____

U.S. and international orders payable in U.S. funds.
Prices are subject to change.

Name: _____

Street: _____

City: _____ Prov./State _____

Country:_____ Zip code _____

Make Cheque or money order payable to: **PicNics Publishing**
P.O. Box 2461, Sechelt
British Columbia, Canada
V0N 3A0

For large volume purchases, contact: **PicNics Publishing.**
Fax: (604) 885-4375
Or fax: 1-800-947-5577

Please allow for 2 - 3 weeks delivery.

KID'S CHOICE
COOKBOOK

ORDER FORM

Order **KID'S CHOICE COOKBOOK** at $14.95 per book
plus $4.00 (total order) for shipping and handling.

Number of books	_____ @ $14.95	=	_____
Postage and handling		=	$ 4.00
Subtotal	_____	=	_____
In Canada add 7% GST	_____	=	_____
Total enclosed	_____	=	_____

U.S. and international orders payable in U.S. funds.
Prices are subject to change.

Name: _____

Street: _____

City: _____ Prov./State _____

Country:_____ Zip code _____

Make Cheque or money order payable to: **PicNics Publishing**
P.O. Box 2461, Sechelt
British Columbia, Canada
V0N 3A0

For large volume purchases, contact: **PicNics Publishing.**
Fax: (604) 885-4375
Or fax: 1-800-947-5577

Please allow for 2 - 3 weeks delivery.